Dear New Cancer Fighter
A Guide for Kids with Leukemia

written by Caleb Cook
illustrated by Estella Patrick

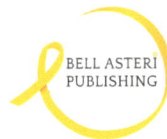

BELL ASTERI
PUBLISHING

Published by Bell Asteri Publishing
209 West 2nd Street #177
Fort Worth TX 76102
www.bellasteri.com

Published in the United States of America

ISBN: 978-1-957604-76-3 (paperback)
ISBN: 978-1-957604-77-0 (hardback)

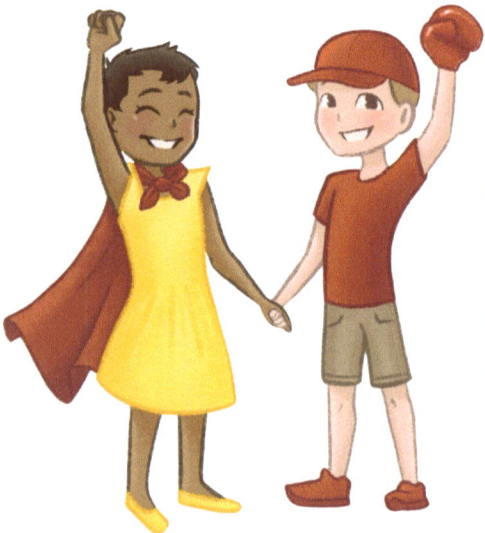

You have been diagnosed with leukemia. I know how you feel. I found out I had leukemia when I was six years old. I know this can be confusing and scary, but doctors and nurses will help you through your journey.

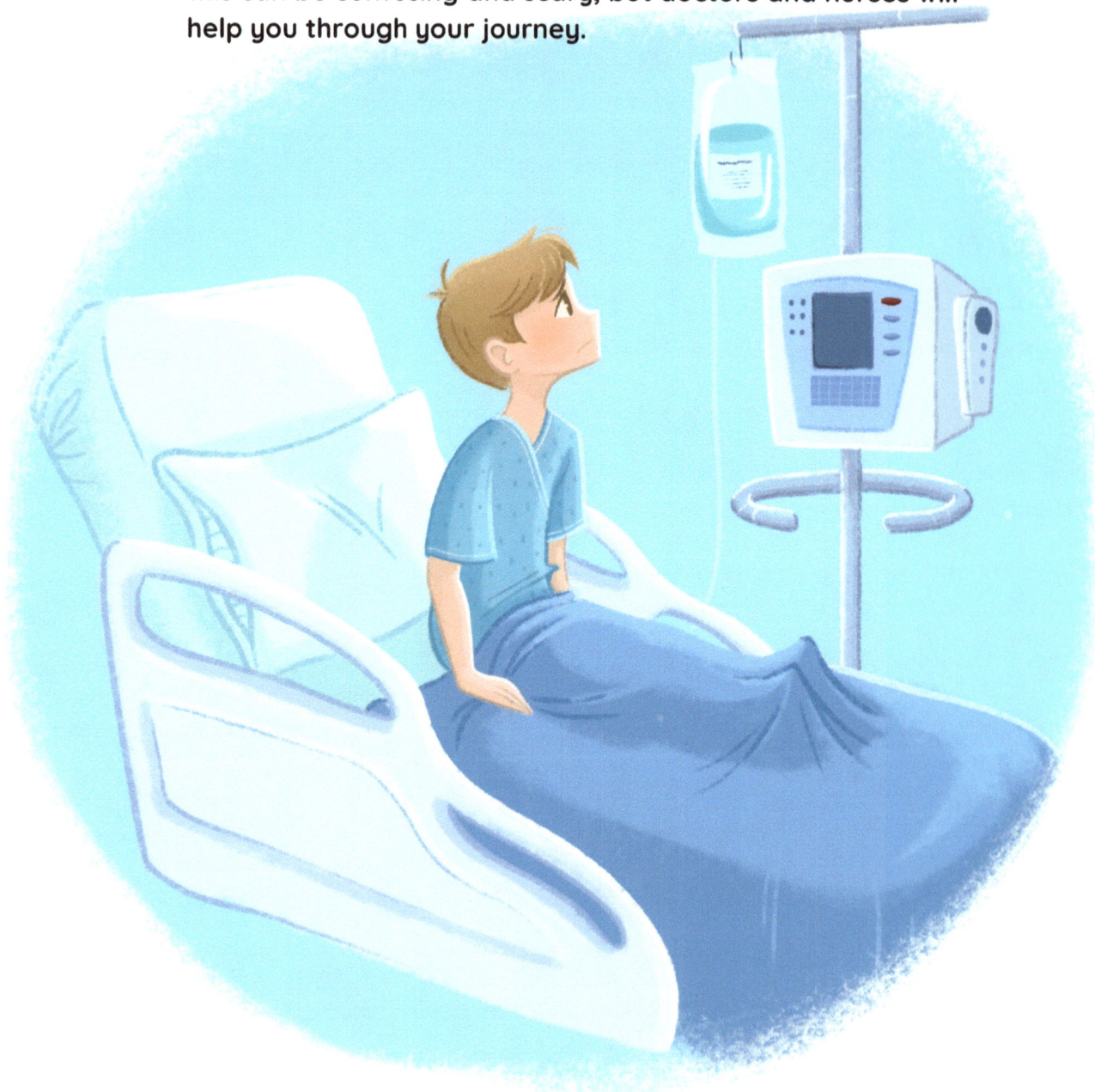

I hope you know that you are not alone! Many kids have been treated for this disease. It is the most common childhood cancer, but the treatments were made to help you get stronger, like they helped me.

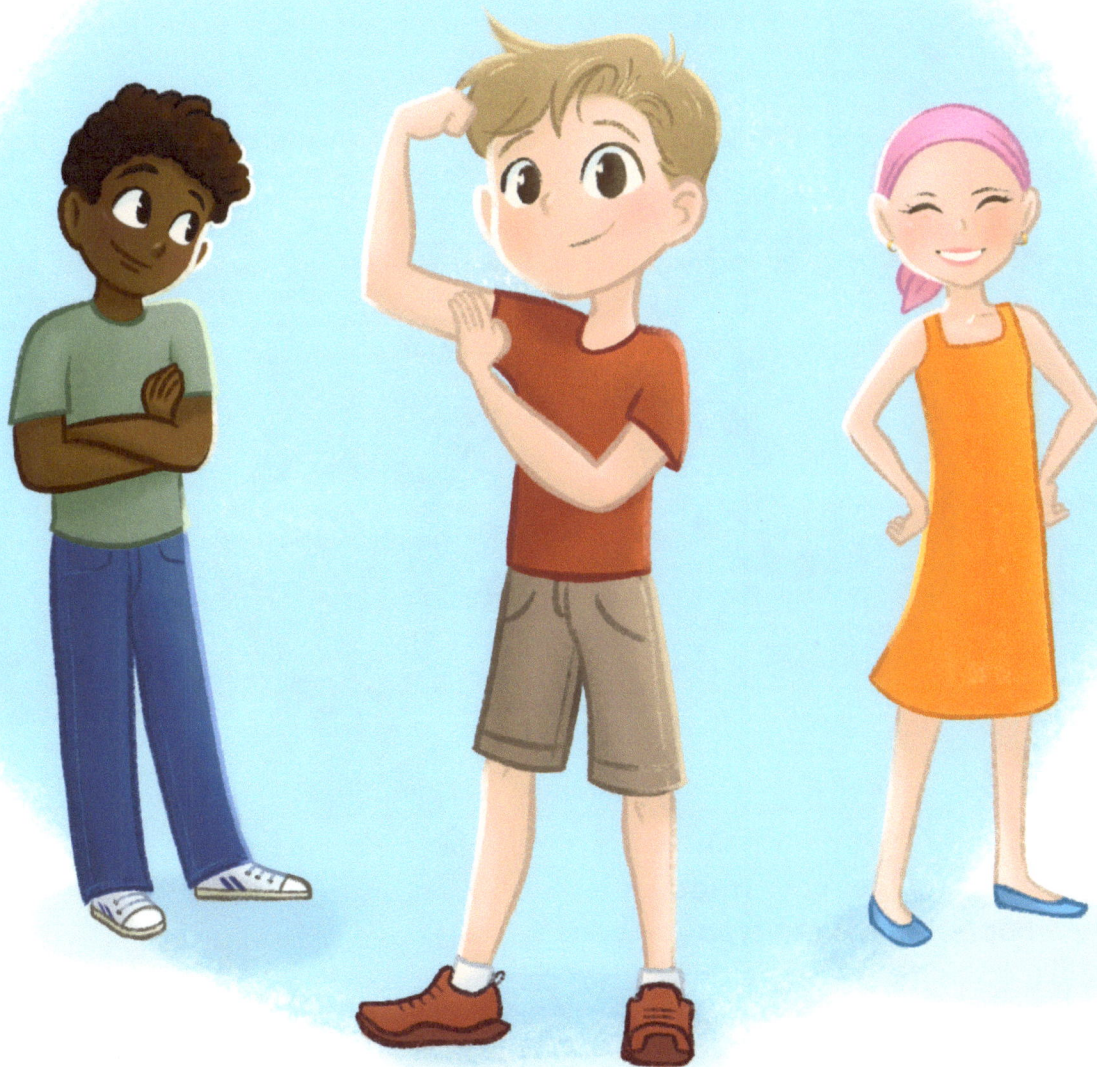

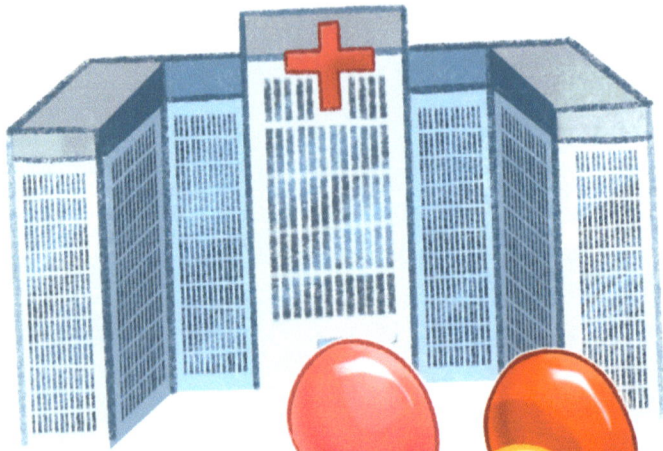

At first, you may spend time in the hospital while your doctors work hard to find the best ways to treat you.

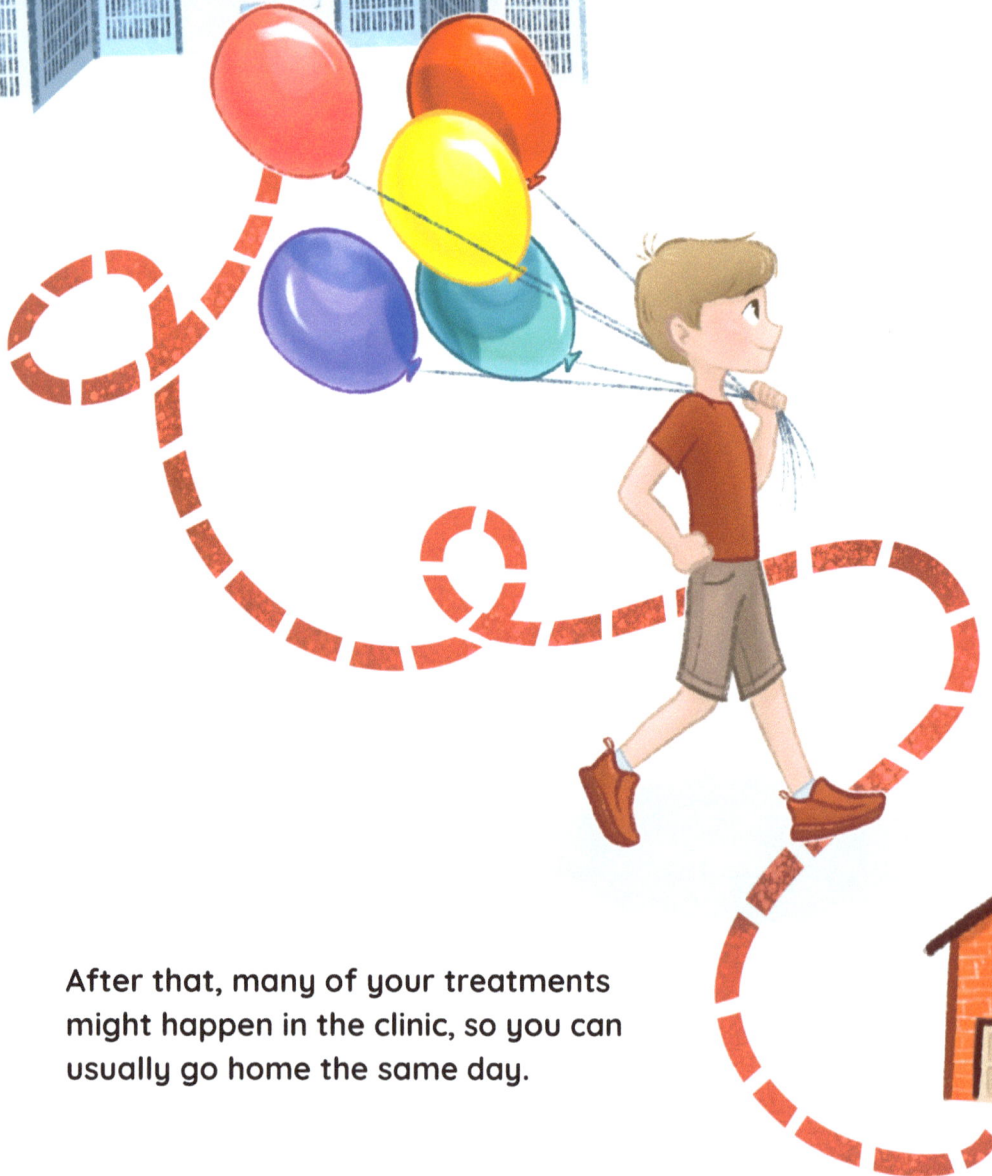

After that, many of your treatments might happen in the clinic, so you can usually go home the same day.

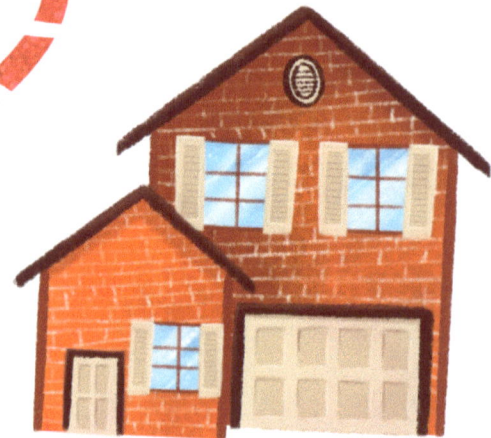

When cancer happens, some cells in your body stop working the right way and take over.

Special medicine called chemotherapy helps fight those bad cells.

Chemo makes them weaker, so you can start feeling better.

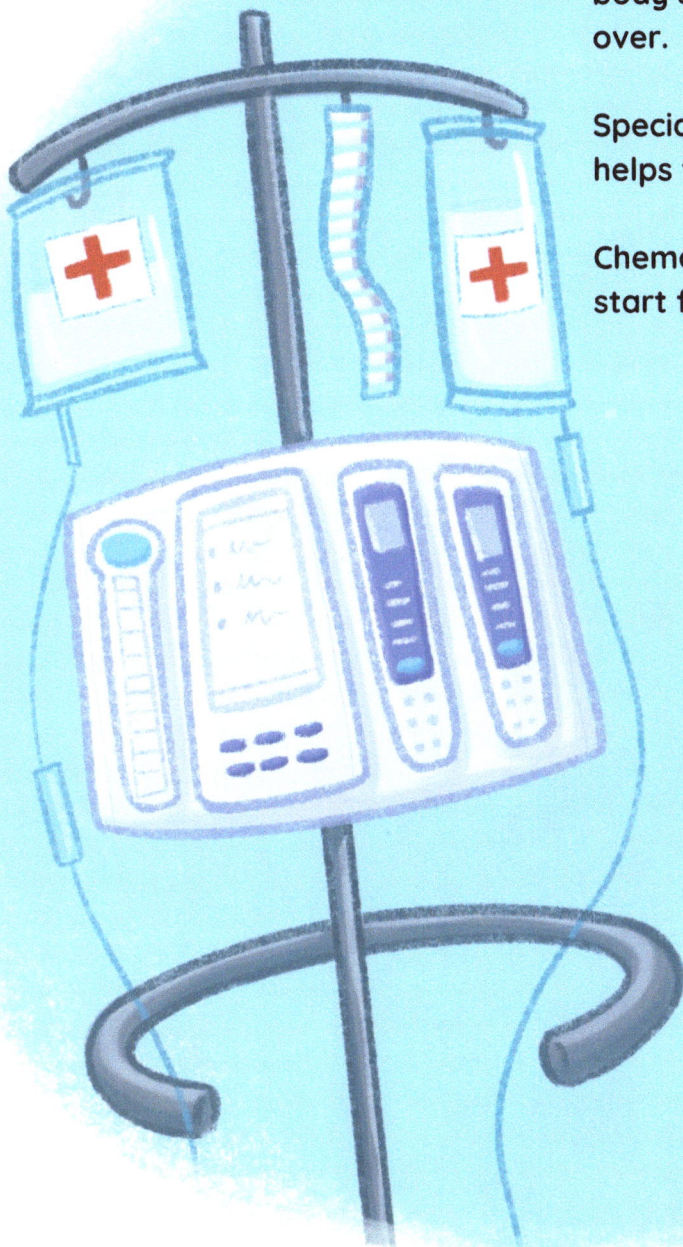

You'll get to meet someone called a child life specialist. They bring fun moments to your day. Look what one of them taught me. She helped me imagine my body as a canvas.

You can try it too!

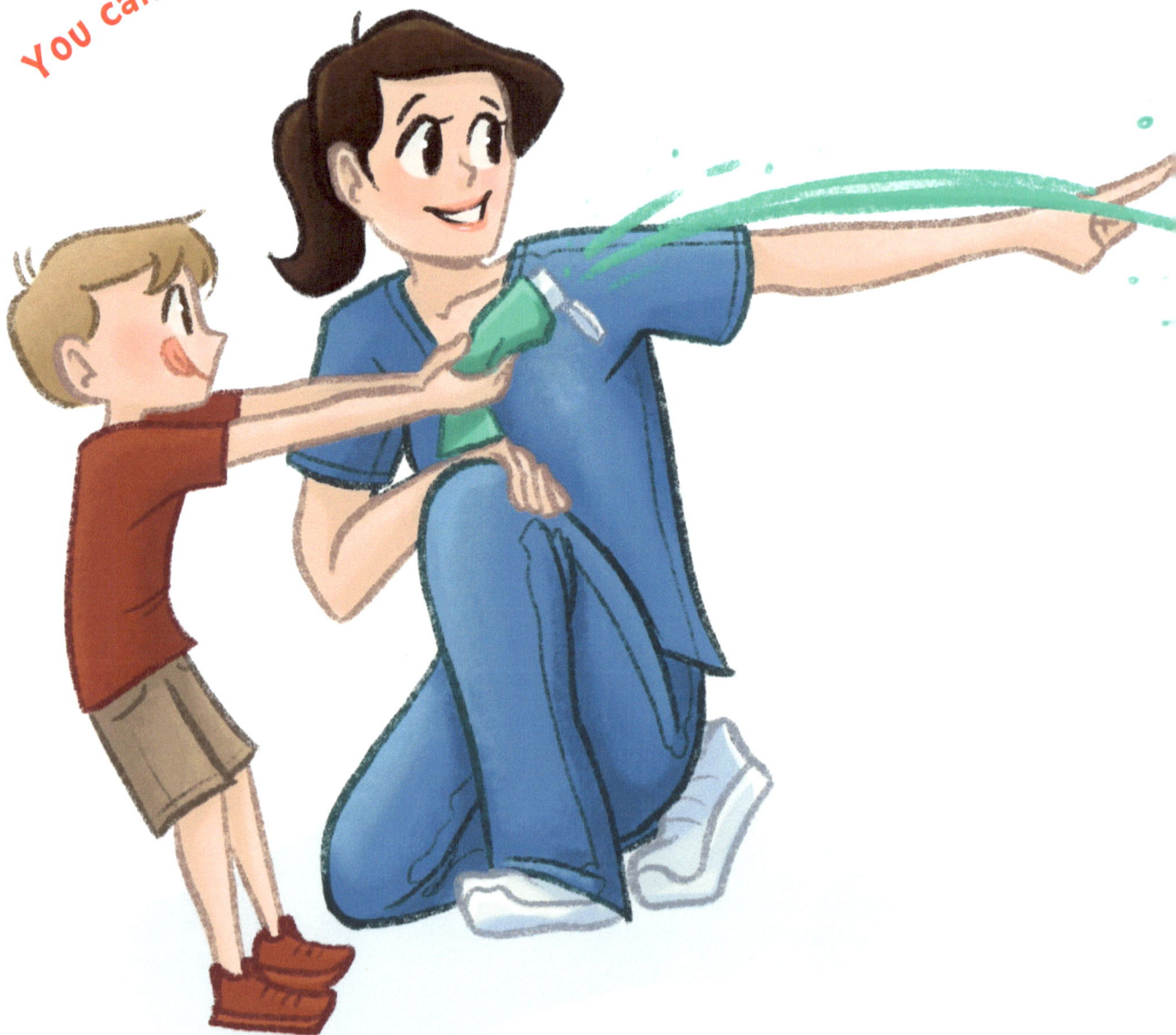

See the orange dots on the paper? They are like cancer cells. When you spray green paint on them, it covers up the orange dots. That's what medicine, like chemotherapy, does inside your body. It destroys the bad cells and lets the healthy ones take over.

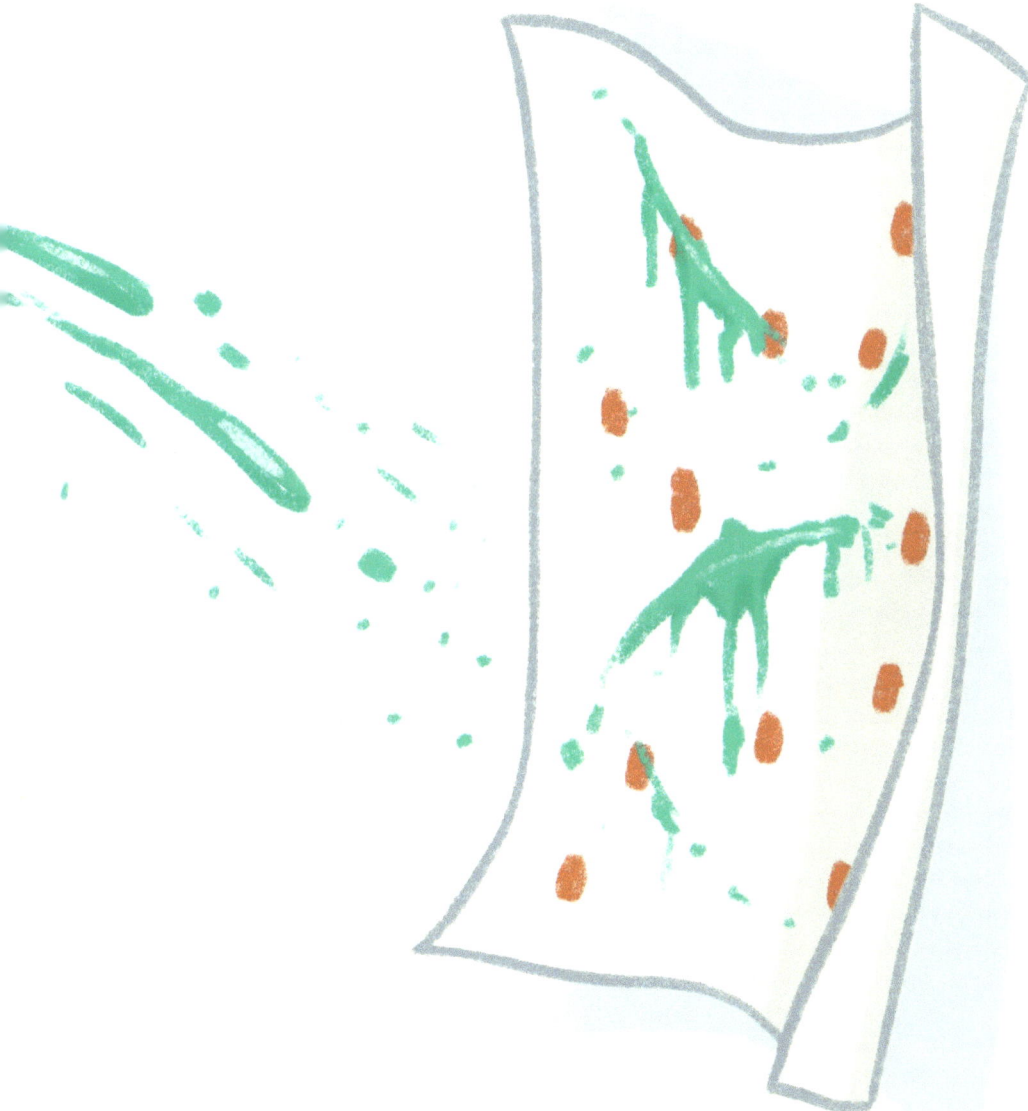

Sometimes you need to swallow medicine to heal your body. I only knew how to swallow food at first, so I took lessons in the hospital.

I started with a tiny sprinkle. Then I worked my way up to bigger pieces of candy. Before long, I could swallow pills. You can learn too!

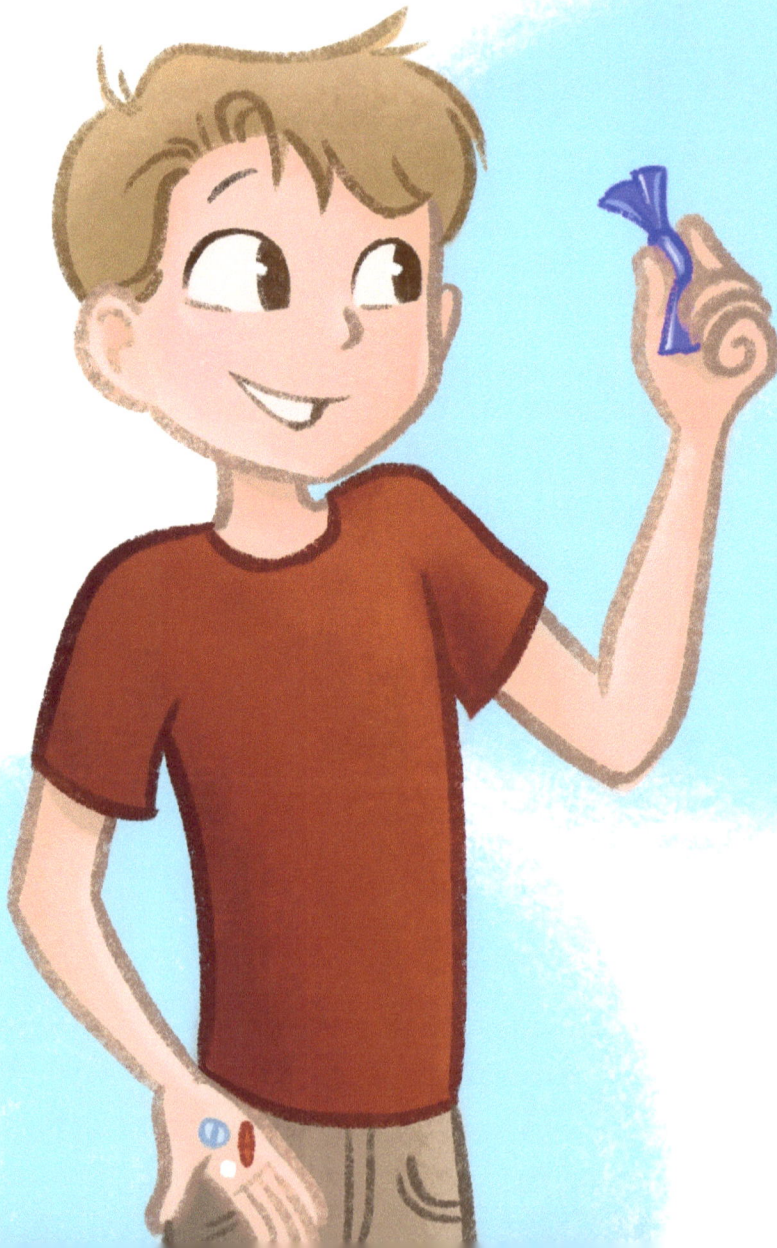

Maybe you can make pill charts, like I did!
I even had blinking lights on one. It made it more exciting.

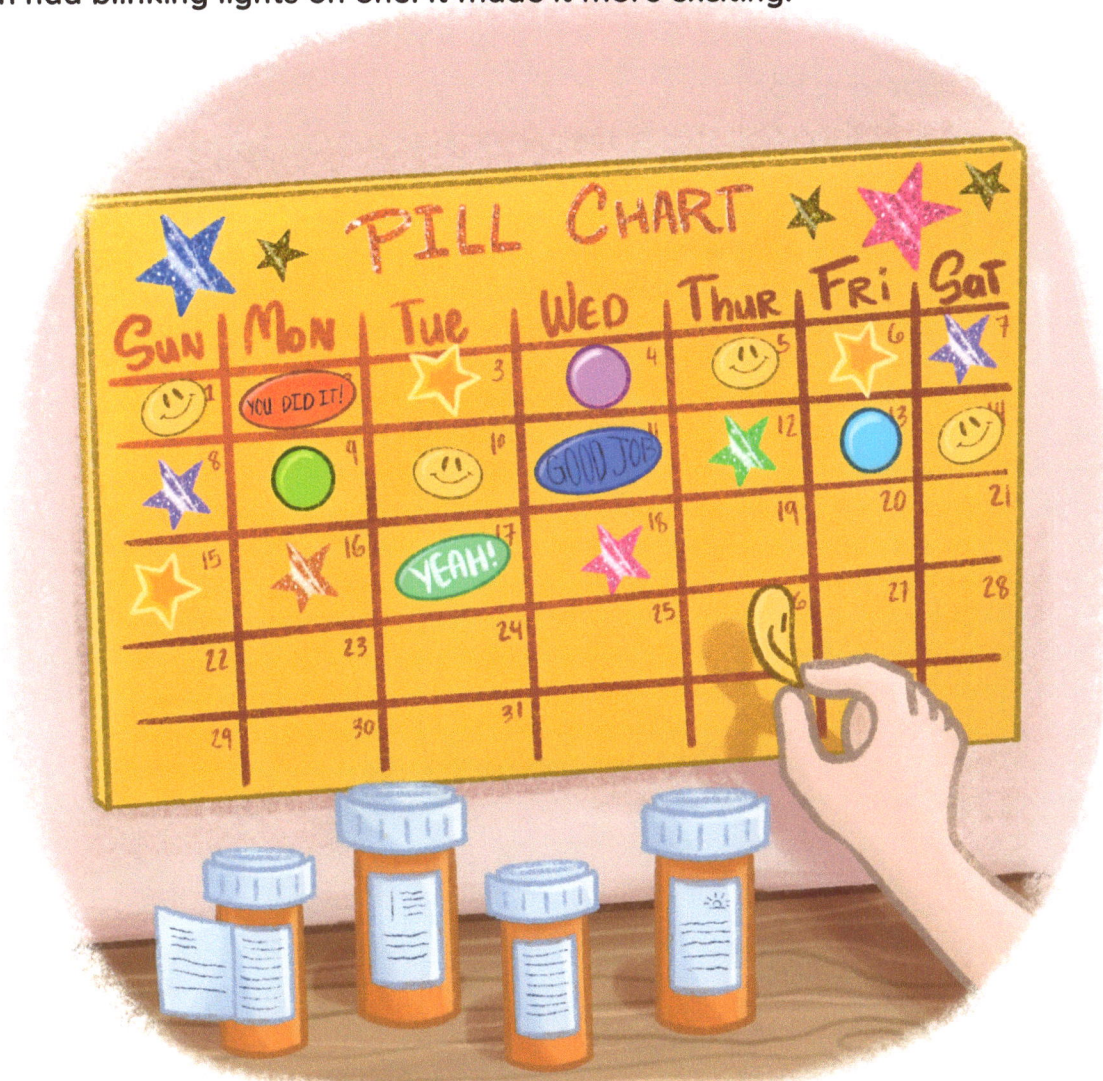

Just remember: Every pill you take is one step closer to
feeling stronger and getting healthier.
YOU'VE GOT THIS!

I have a lot of fun memories from the hospital! Volunteers would come by in silly costumes to visit my room.

Sometimes they sang songs or put on playful puppet shows.

I bet they make you smile, too!

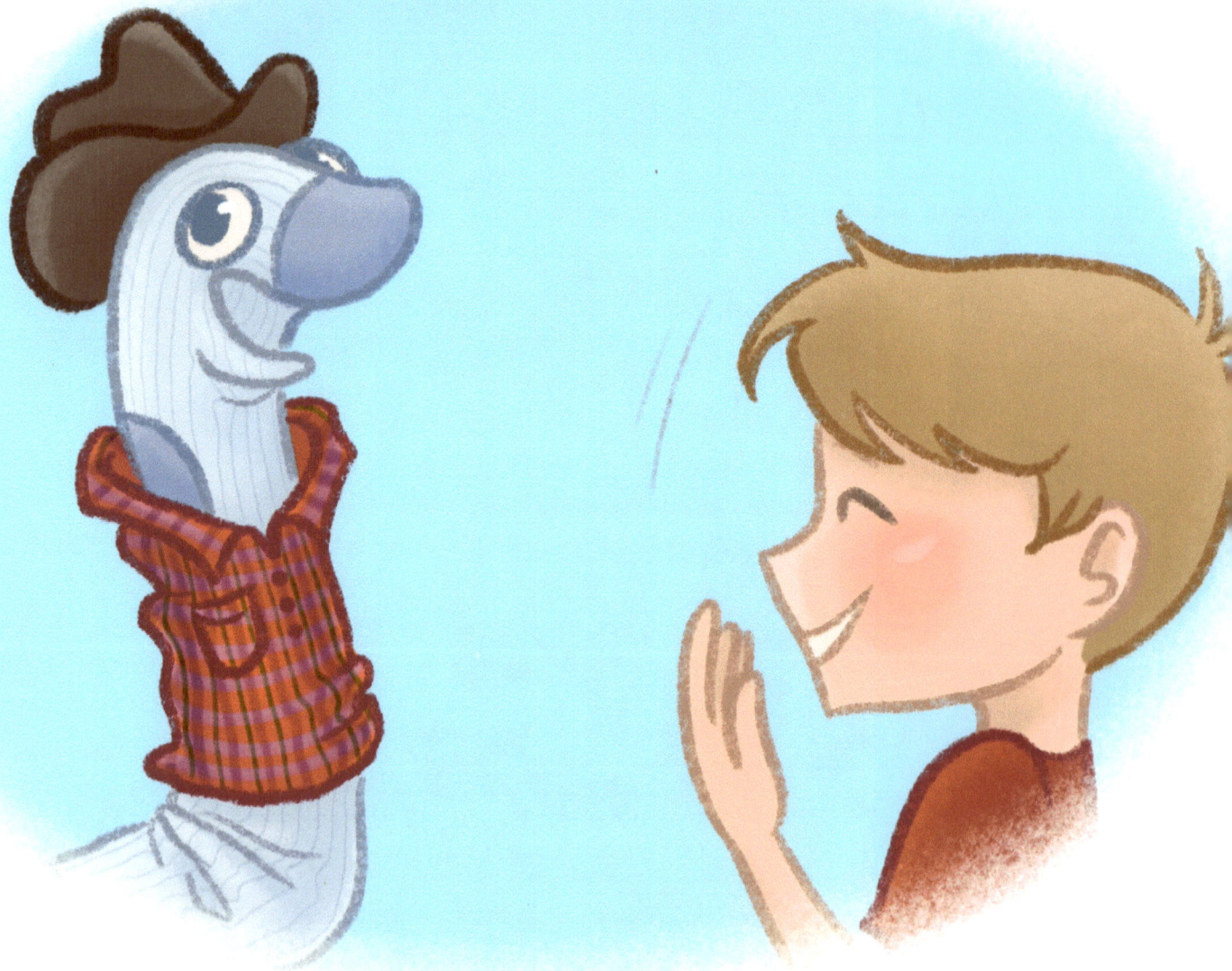

When I was feeling strong, I visited an exciting place called Radio Lollipop in the hospital and got to play games.

It was a nice break to leave my hospital room.

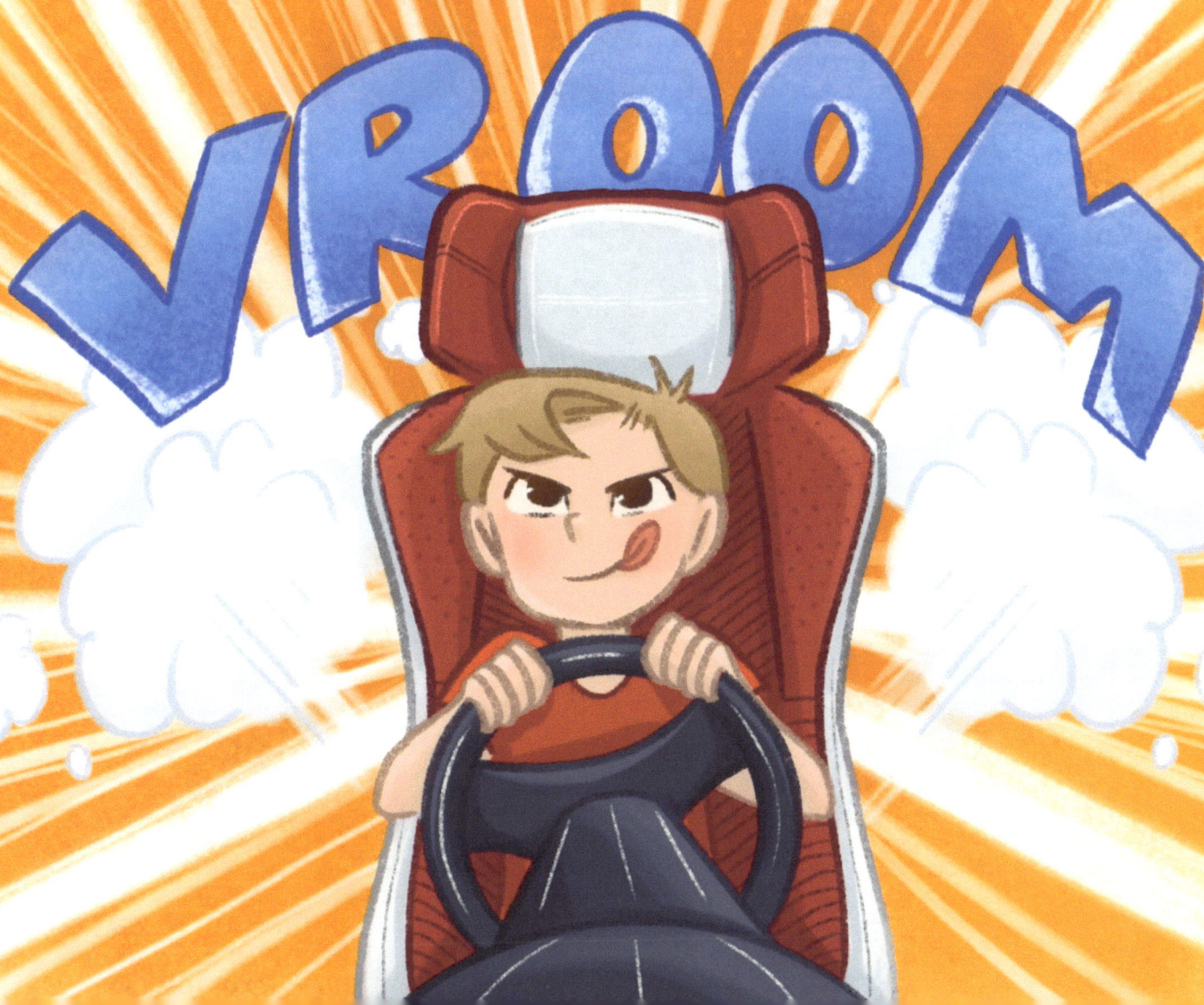

You'll get to do a lot of crafts during your appointments. One time, I painted this cow.

You can paint or color anything you want!

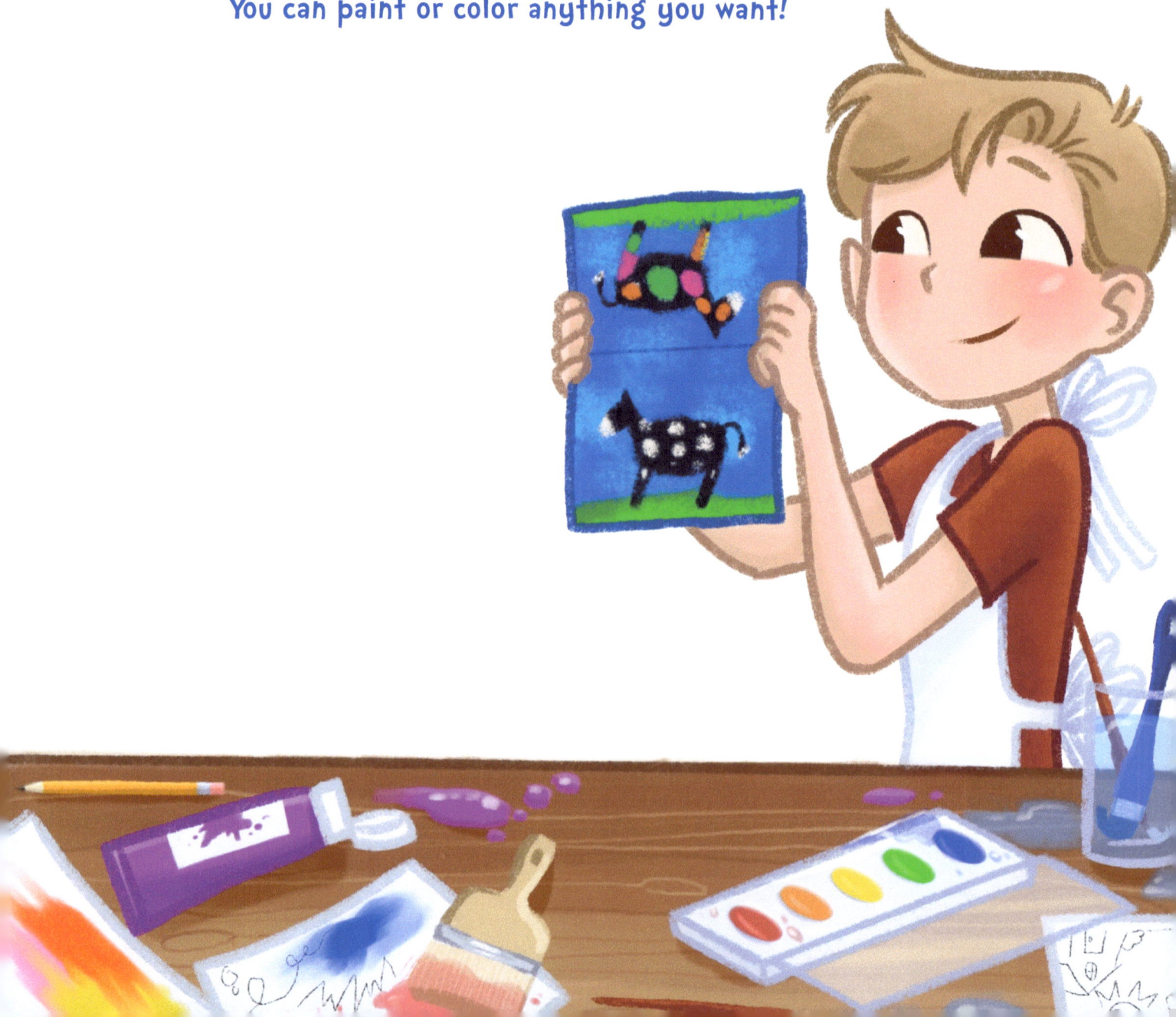

A hospital worker entered my painting into a contest at the Houston Livestock Show and Rodeo, and I won!
That meant I got to ride in a firetruck at the rodeo to celebrate.

They even gave me a cash prize, and guess what?

I got to buy a brand-new toy!

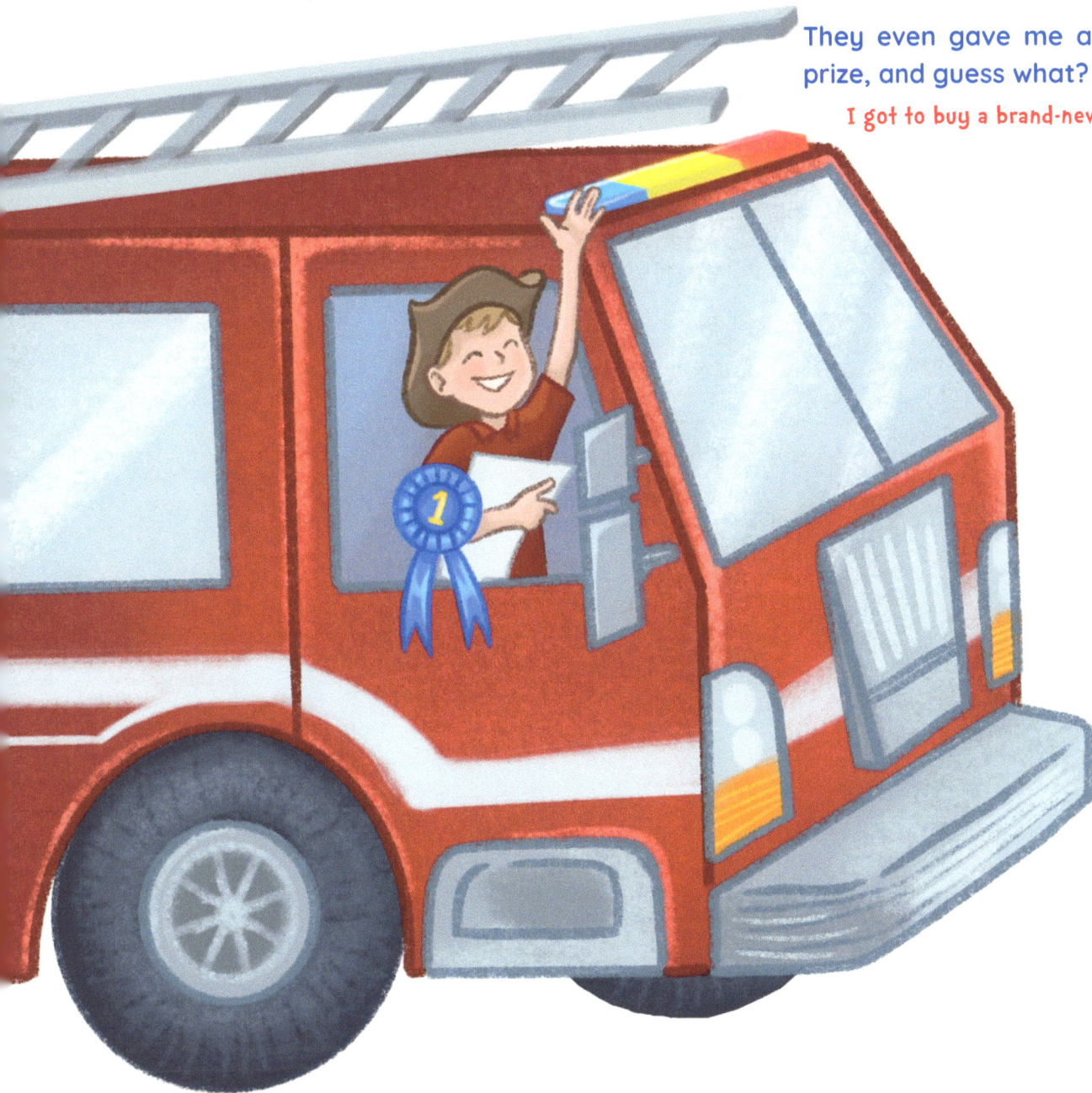

There are many chances to go to fun camps. Sometimes your family gets to go with you, and it's free! Other kids are going through treatments too, so they understand how you're feeling.

It helped my life feel normal again.

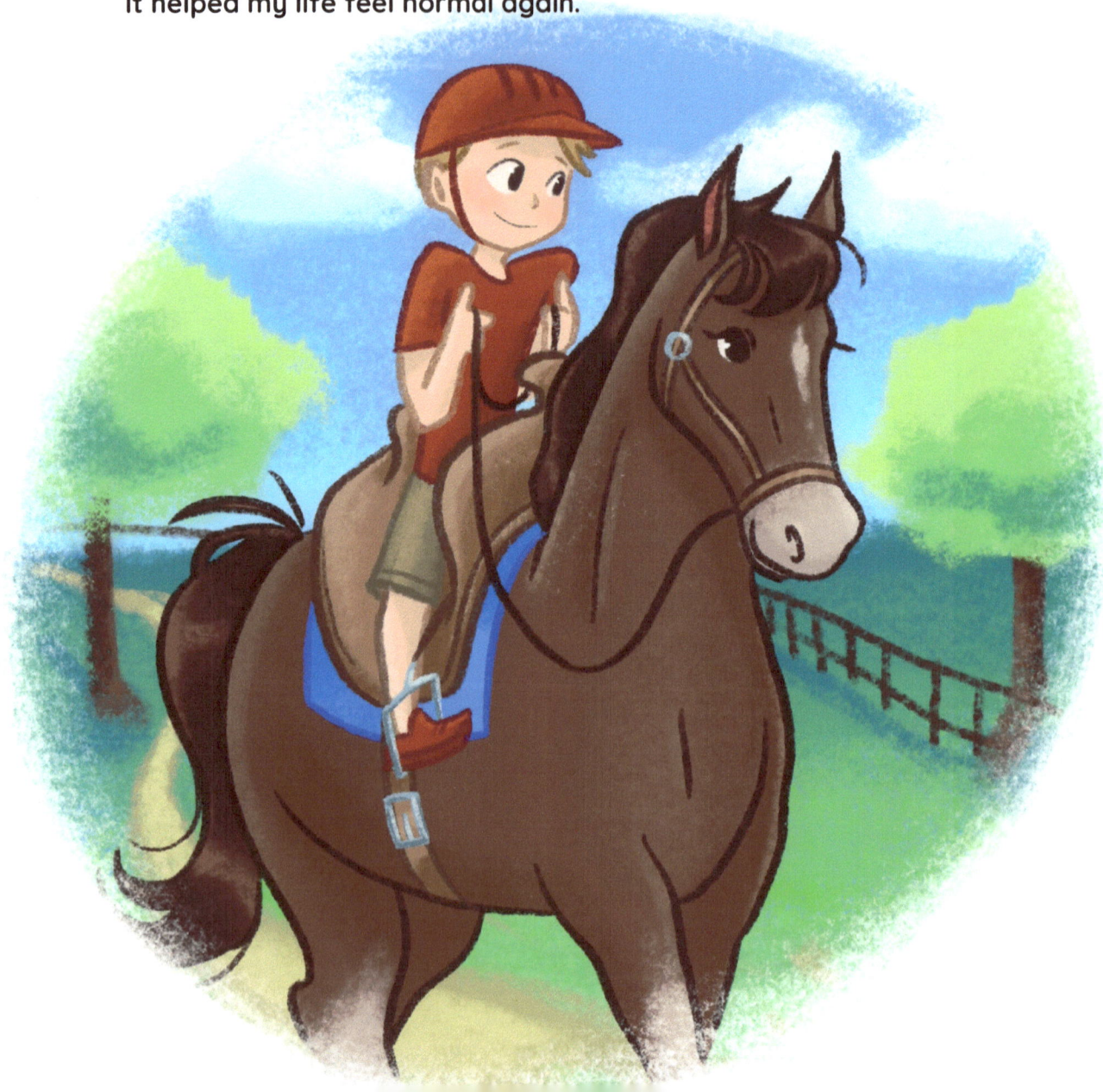

I learned how to ride a horse, climb a rock wall, and even zipline at camp! I still can't believe I could do those things, but I did, and you can too.

These amazing experiences were made possible through special groups like the Periwinkle Foundation and Candlelighters Childhood Cancer Family Alliance.

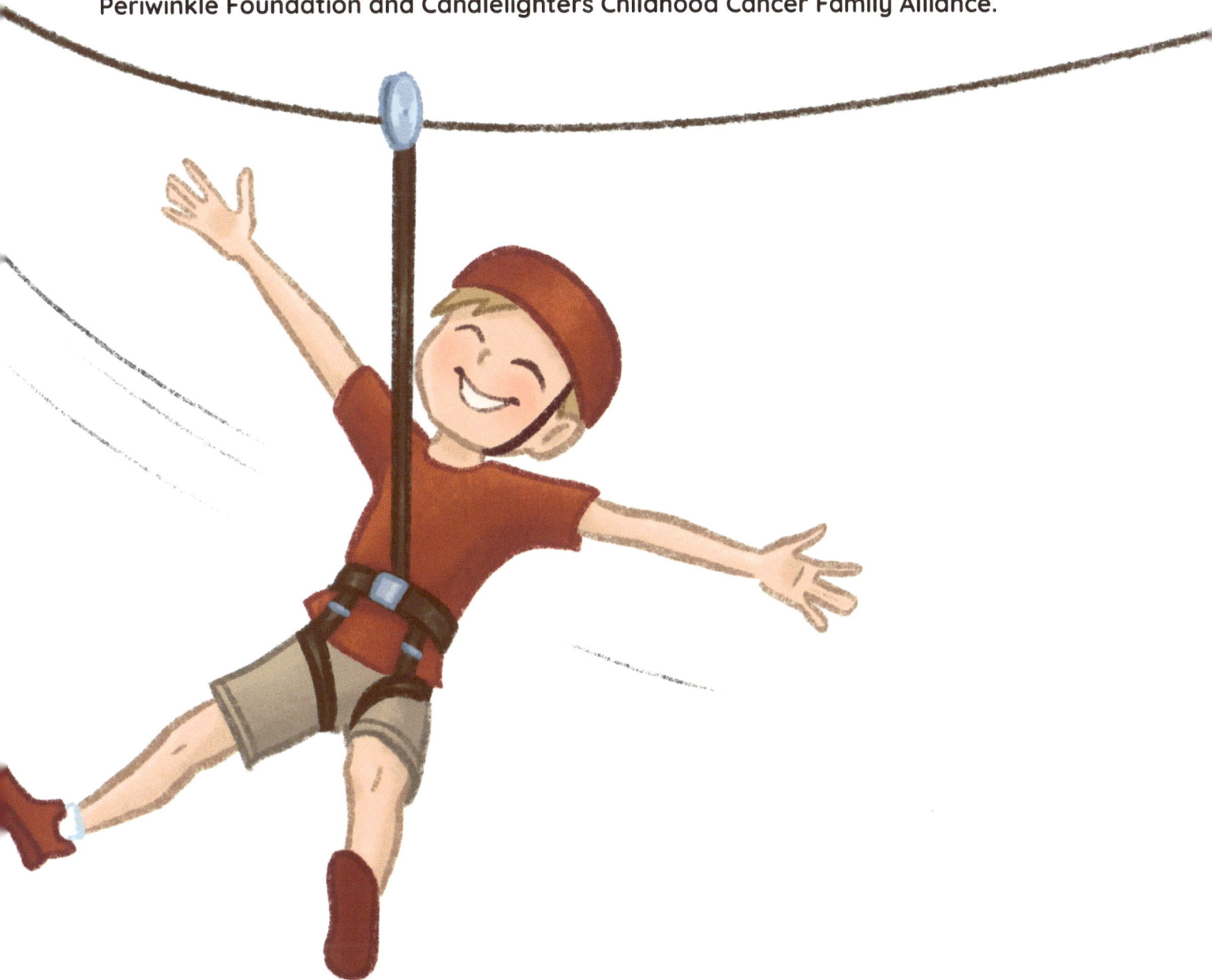

One of the hardest things was losing my hair. Not every kid goes through that, but it helps to understand why it happens. There are ways to make it fun.

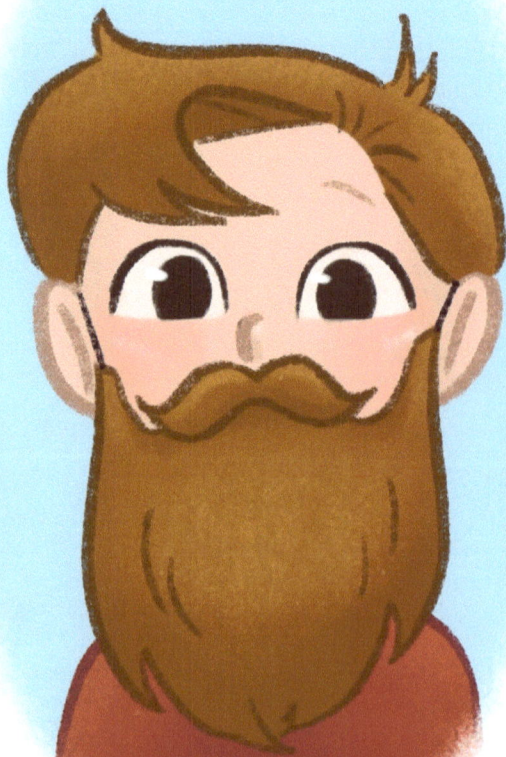

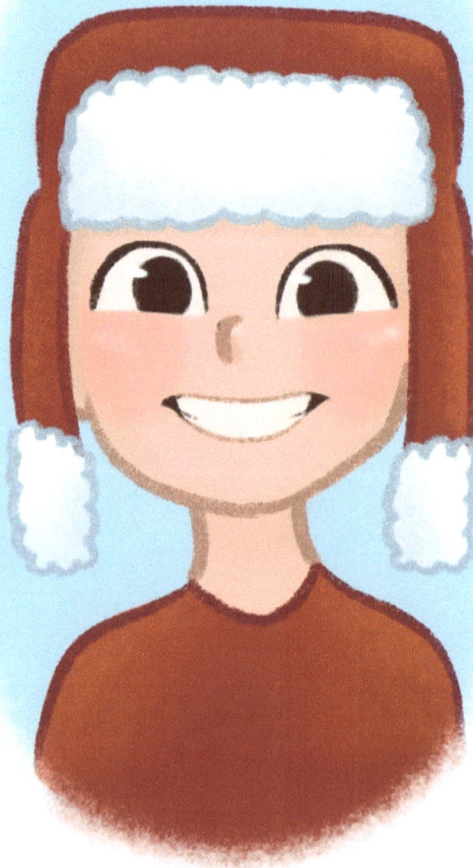

Your medicine is powerful and attacks fast-growing cancer cells. Since your hair also grows fast, it can get affected.

I wore lots of hats and bright, funny wigs. They made me feel better. Plus, they kept my head warm during the winter!

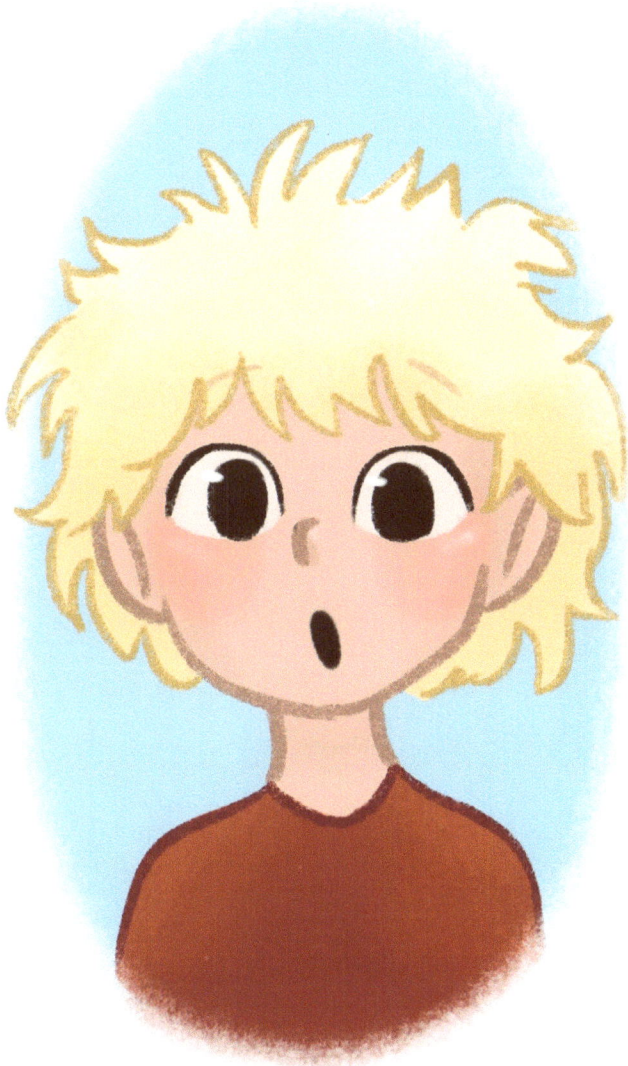

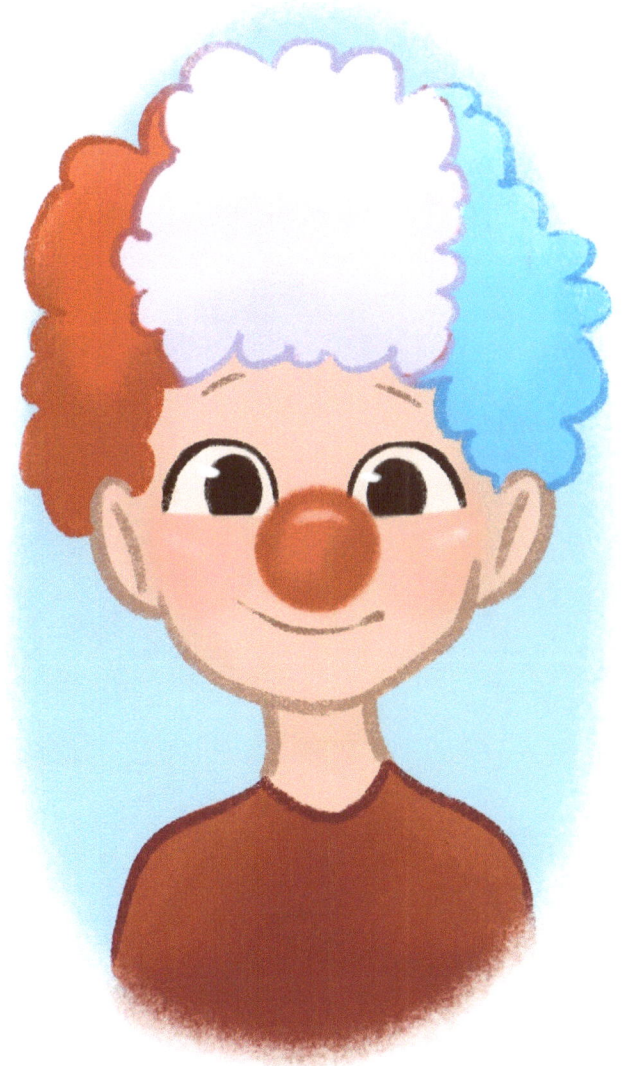

When I first started my treatments, I needed to be extra careful about germs, so I went to school at home instead. I got to pick my own schedule.

I took lots of playtime breaks and ate yummy snacks.

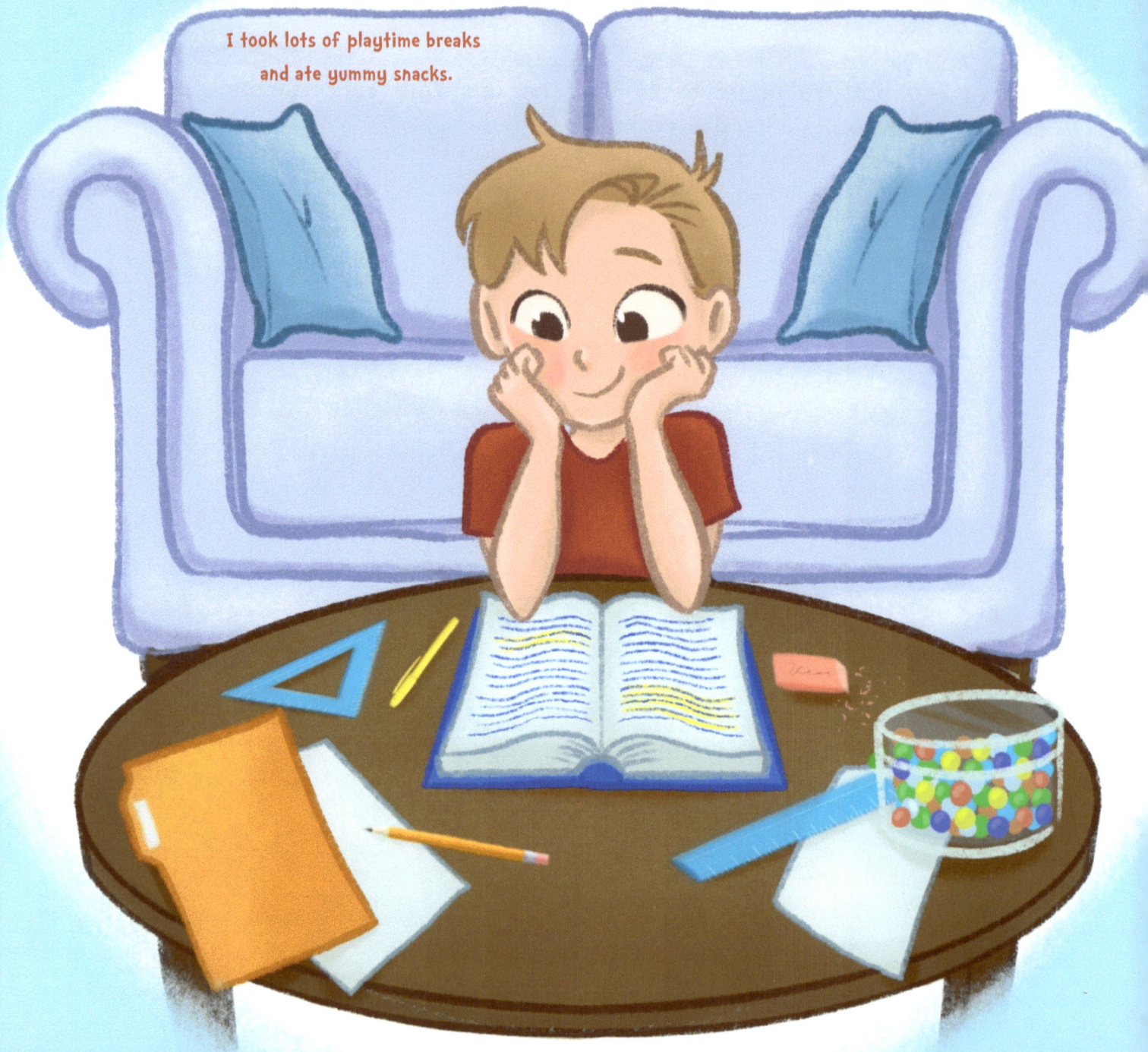

My older brother helped me a lot. We made paper airplanes, and he always made me laugh! I found out later that cancer can be really hard on brothers and sisters, too.

They also need extra love during this time.

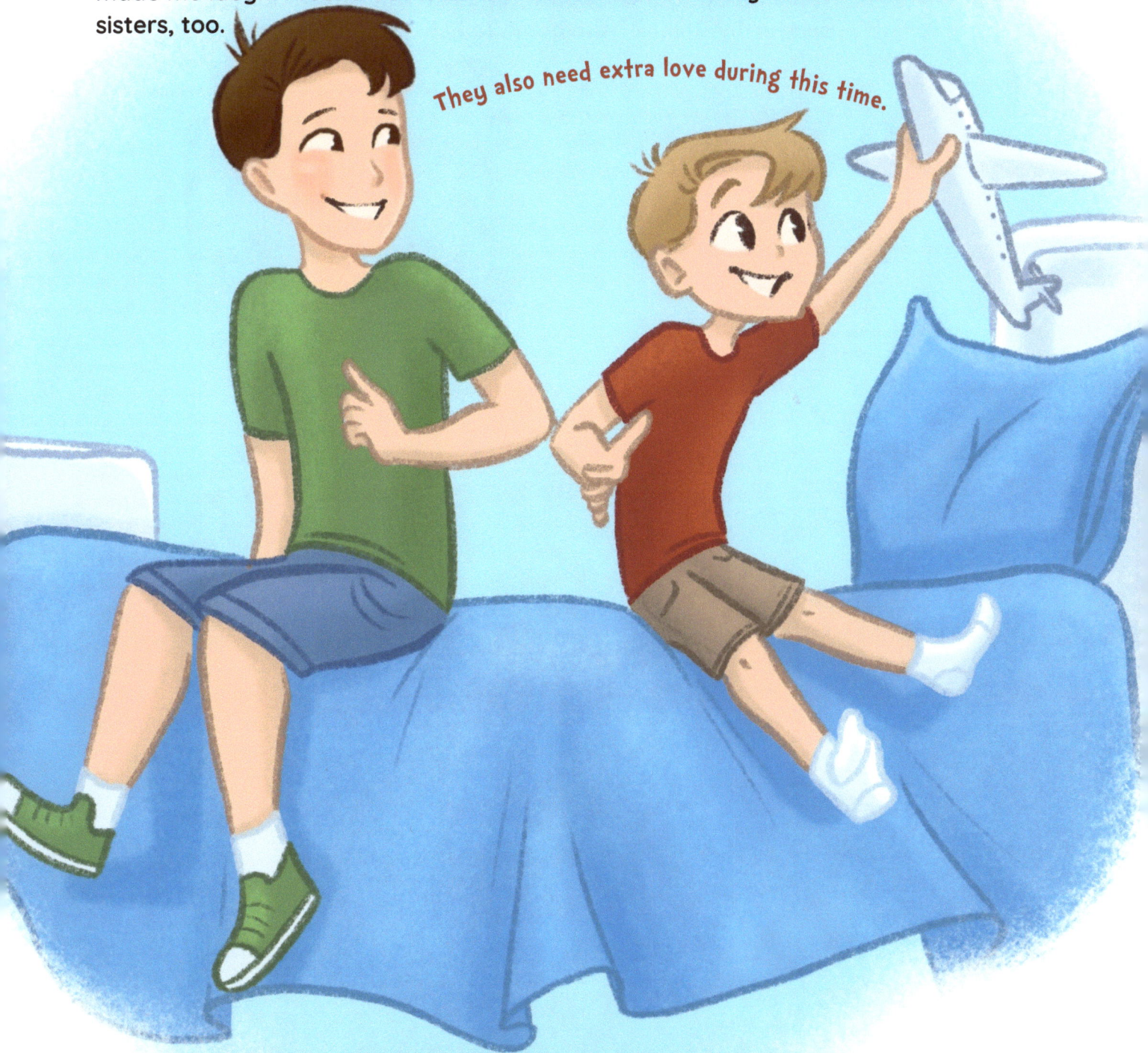

When I went to the hospital for chemotherapy, I always brought comforting things from home to help me feel better.

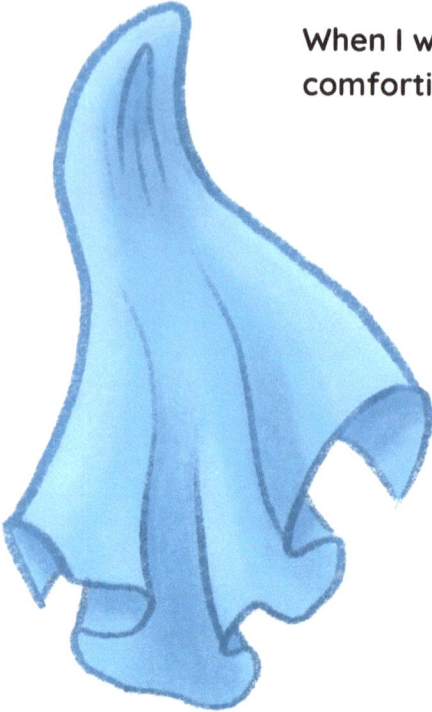

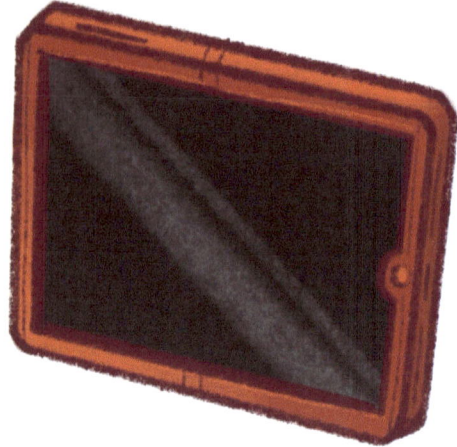

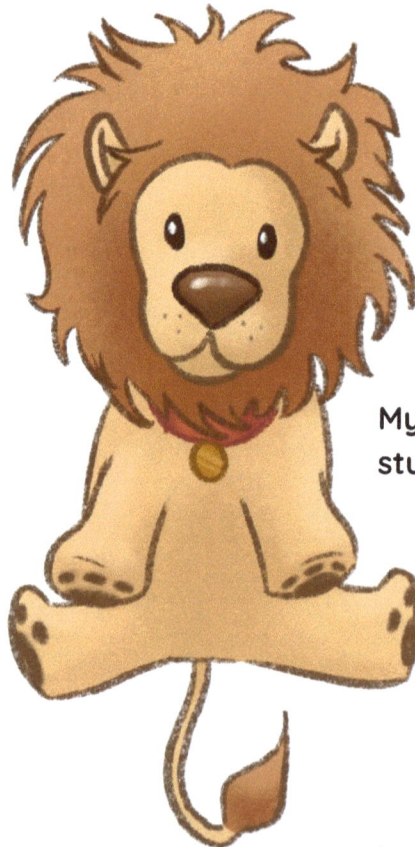

My favorites were a soft blanket, stuffed animals, and my iPad.

At the start of my treatment, I had surgery to get a port inserted. A port is a small device under the skin in the upper chest area. It helps nurses give chemotherapy more easily, so that you don't need needlesticks in your arm each time you have a treatment.

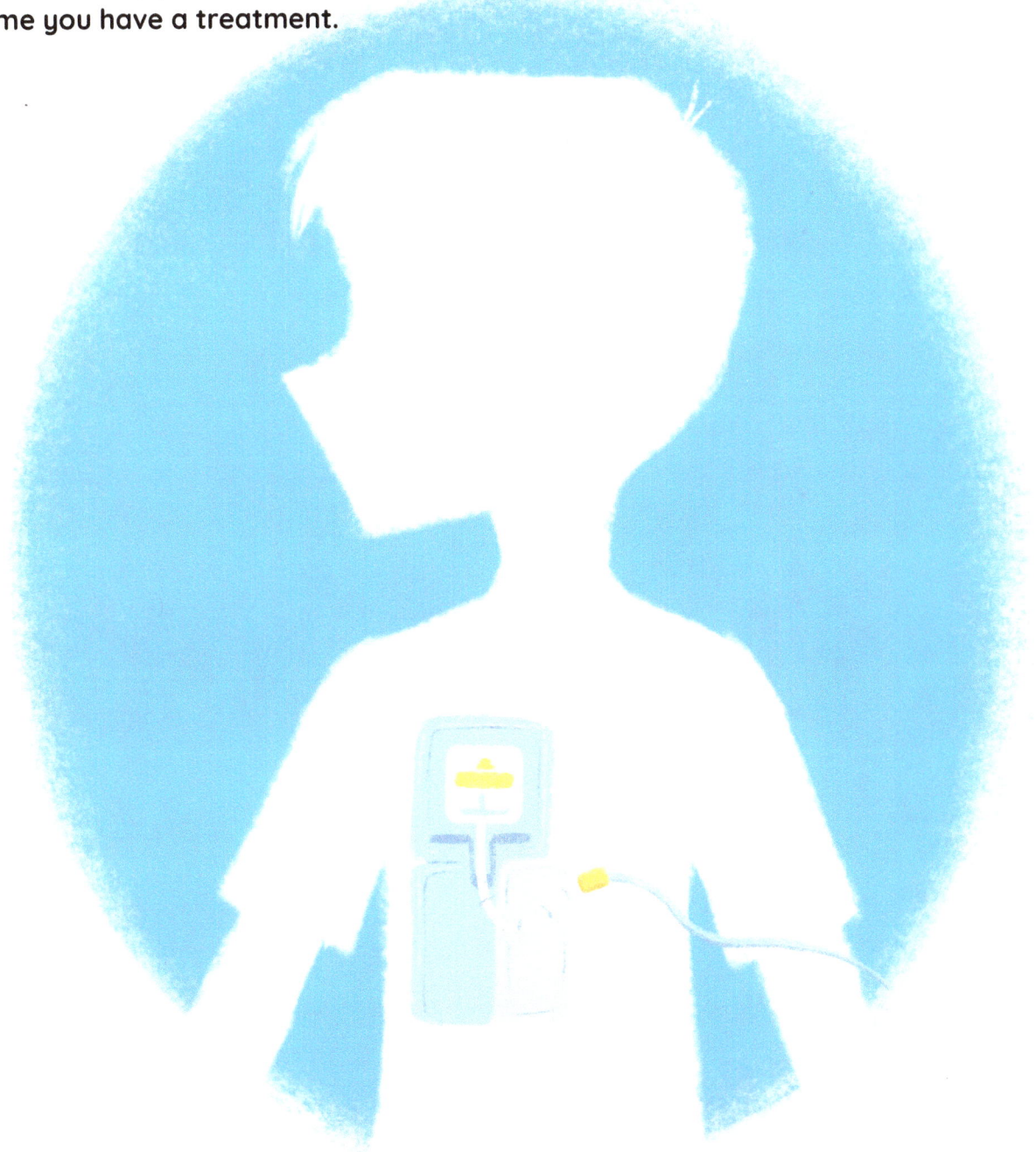

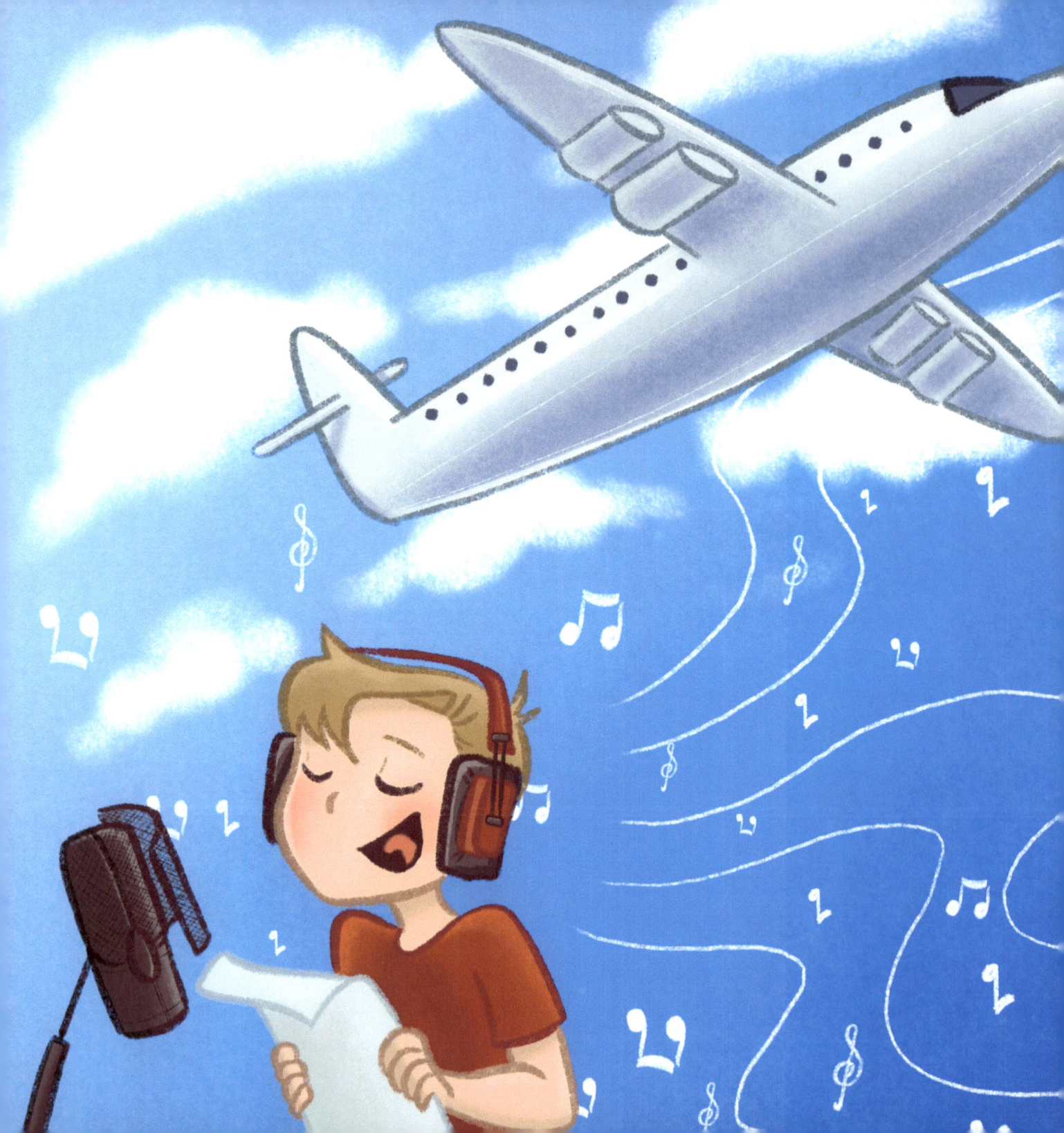

You might get to become a rock star at the hospital. I got to write and record my very own song with a music producer. The studio was called **PURPLE SONGS CAN FLY** because songs are sent flying into the sky and into space by pilots and astronauts.

I wrote mine about football because my dream was to play football when I got stronger. And guess what? I did!

Scan the QR code to listen.

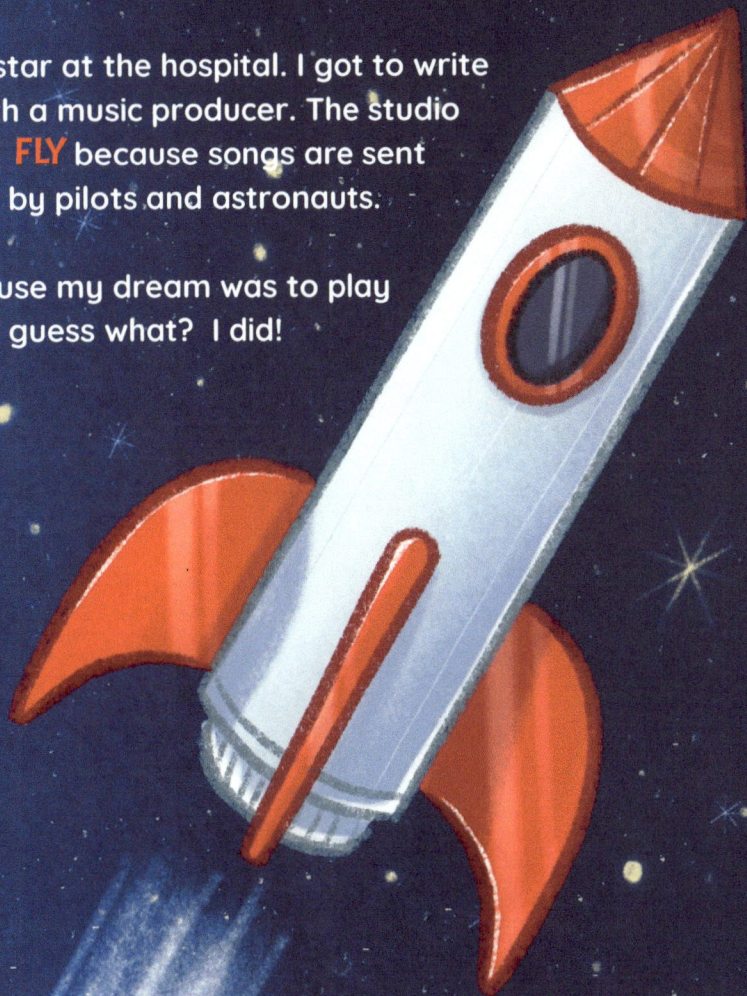

If one of your treatments involves a medicine called steroids, get ready because they can cause the silliest cravings. Look at this...

Can you believe I craved mayonnaise right out of the jar?

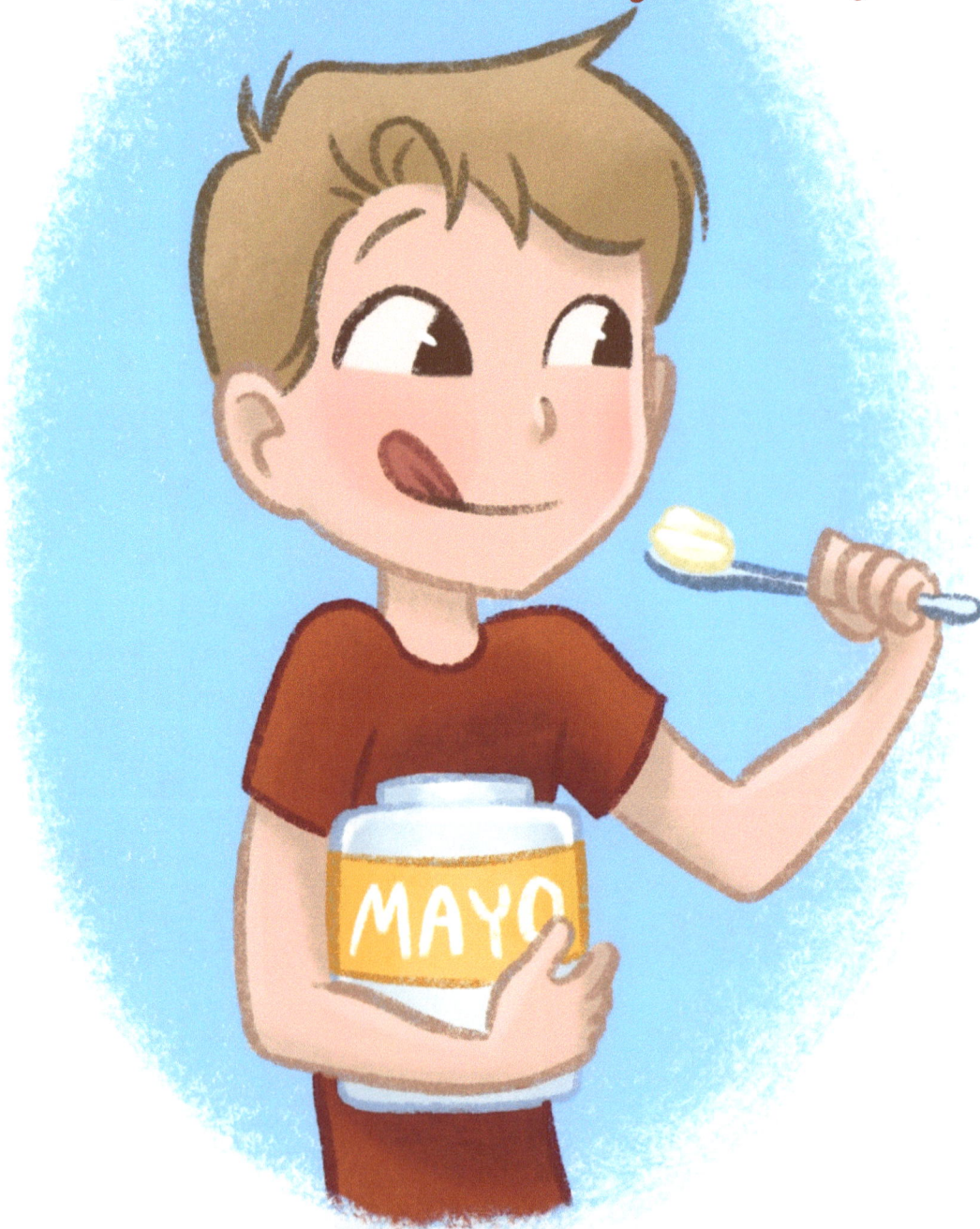

Sometimes I had to get X-rays. I stood really still while they took special pictures to look inside my body. Don't worry! There's nothing to be scared of. And the best part? You don't even have to smile for these pictures.

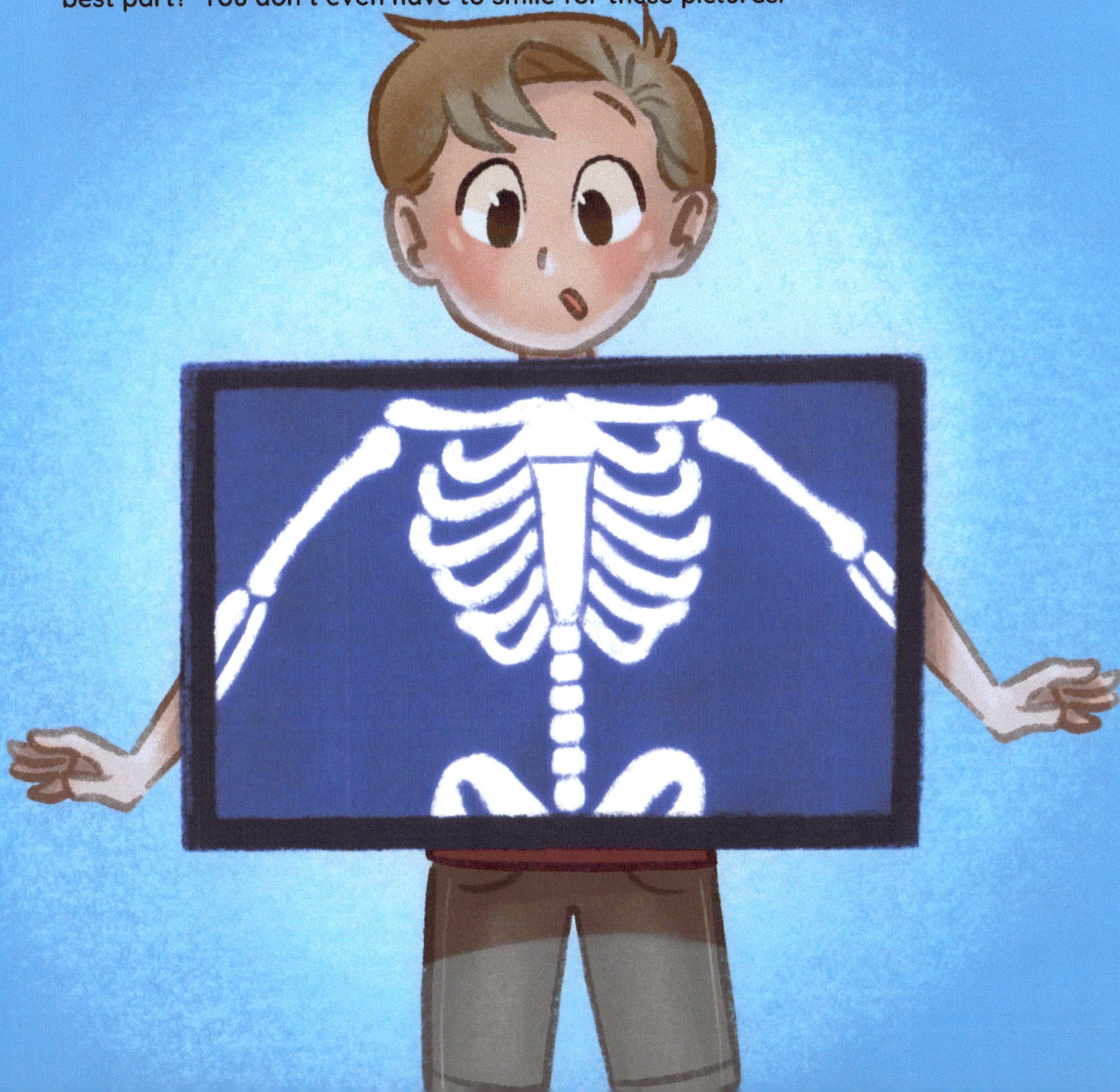

You can usually stay active during treatment, sometimes even work out or play sports!

There were many times when I still got to play baseball. It felt great to be out on the field.

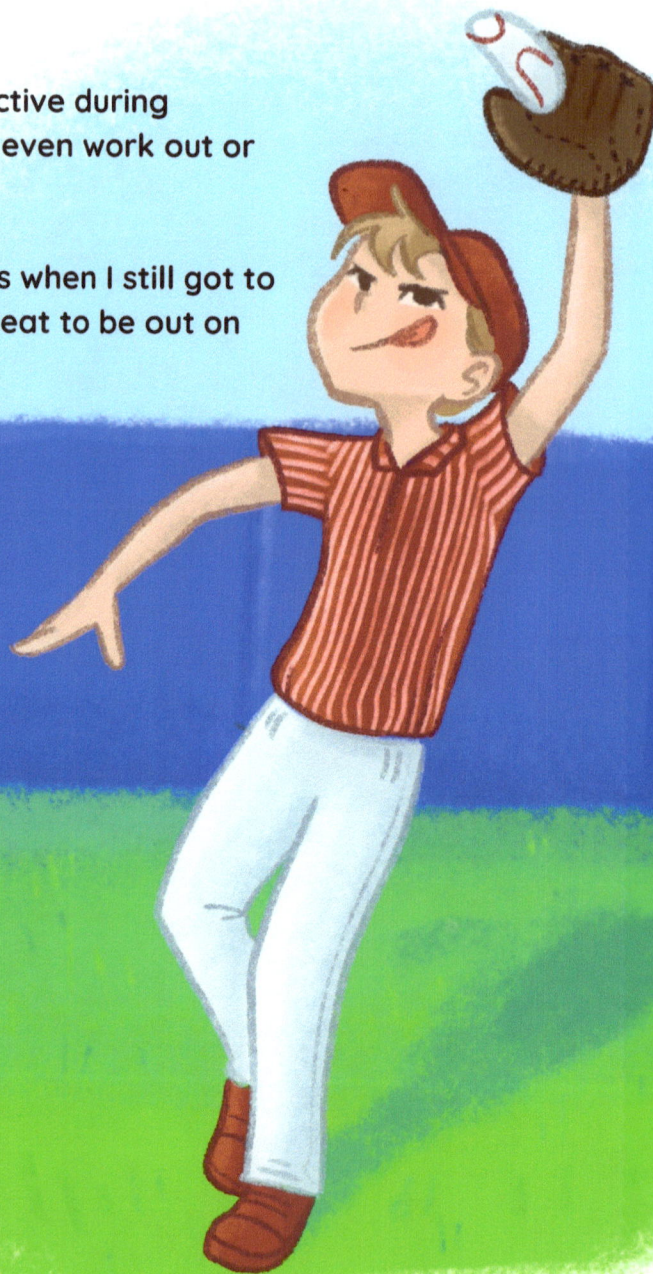

Thanks to several cancer foundations, like the Sunshine Kids, I got to meet amazing, famous athletes. It was such a fun part of my journey!

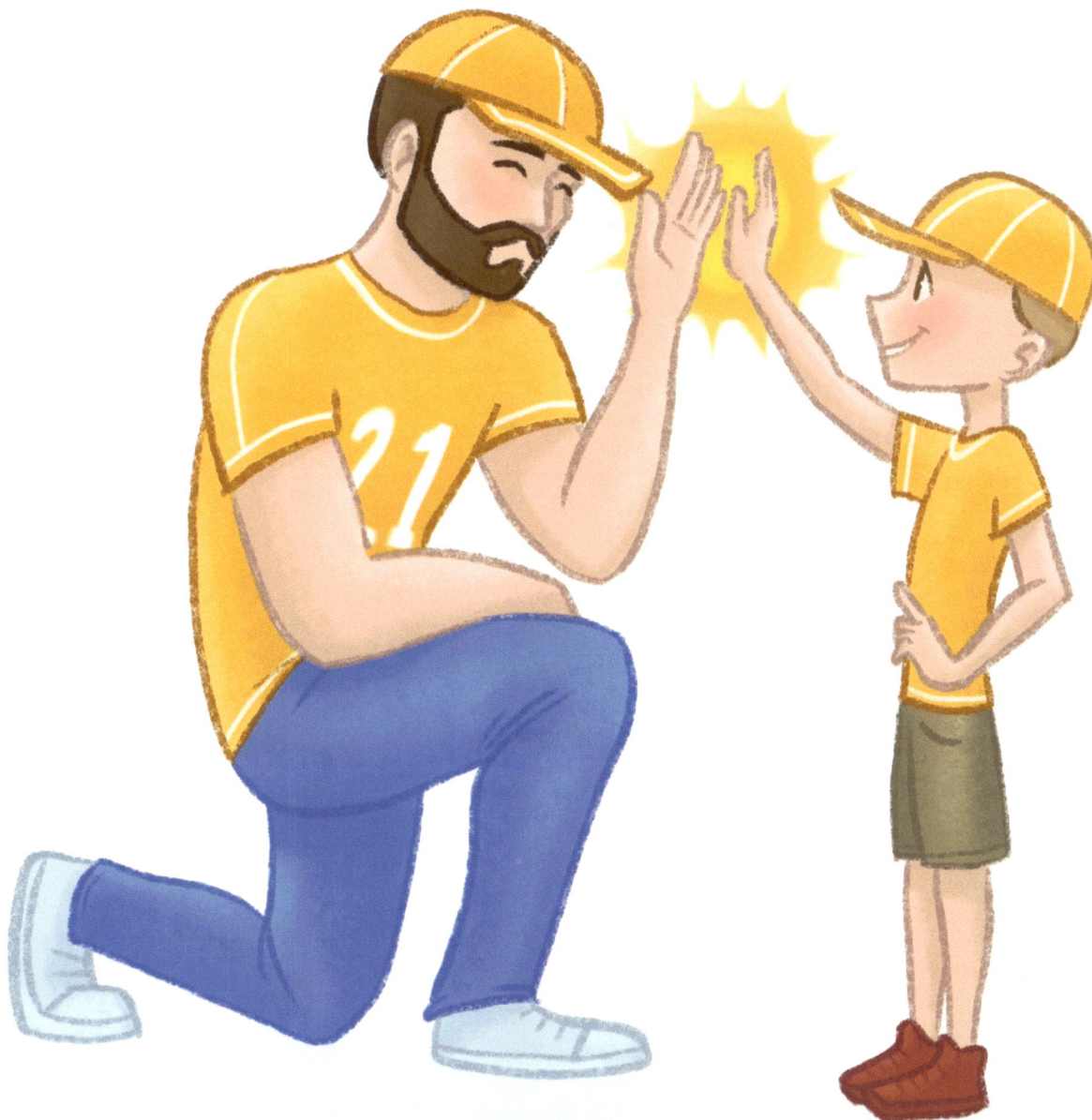

There's a special event called Light The Night. You can carry a glowing lantern and help light up the city. Your loved ones cheer you on. It's a night full of hope, strength, and celebration to raise money for Blood Cancer United, which helps scientists discover even better cancer treatments.

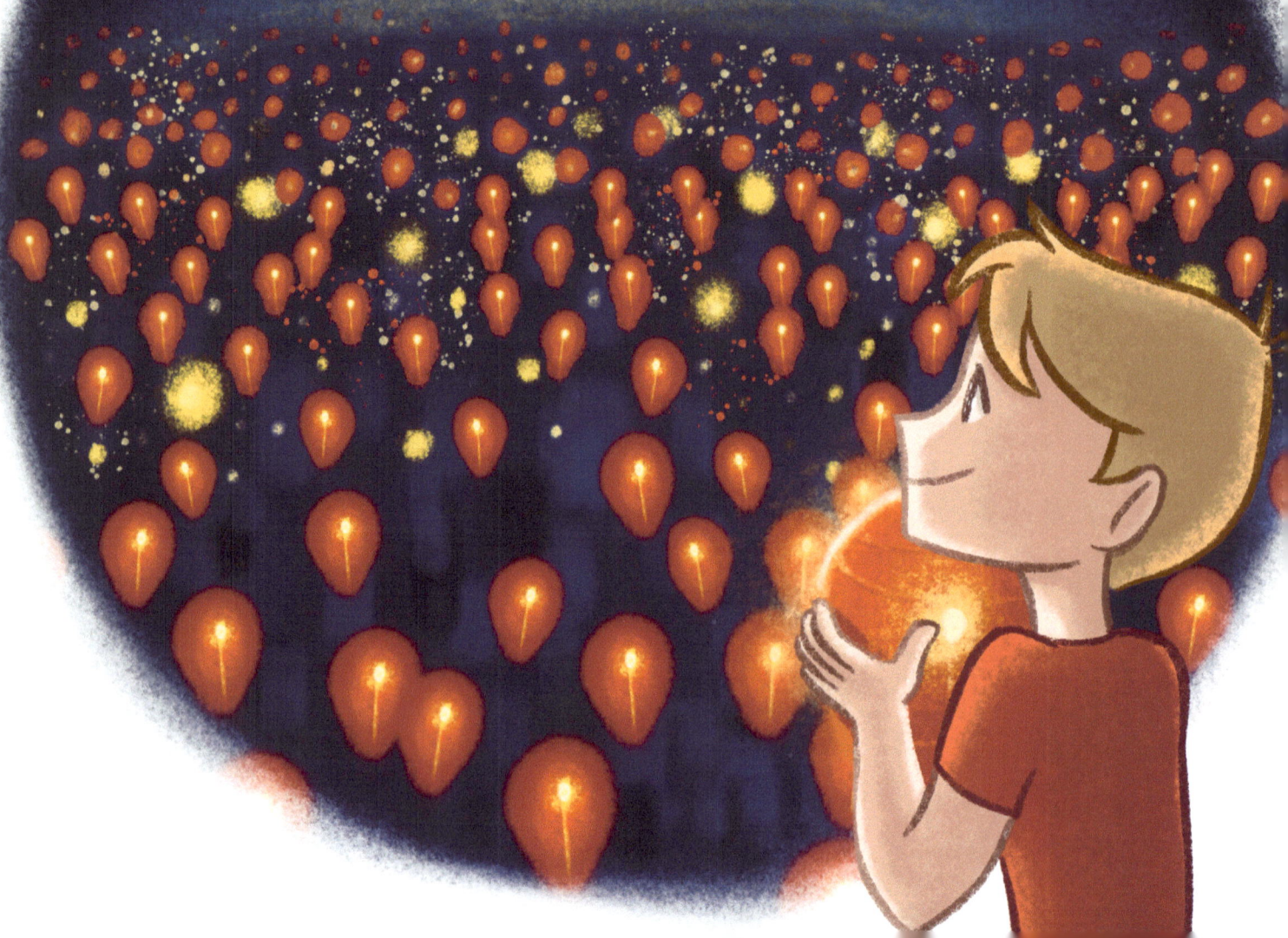

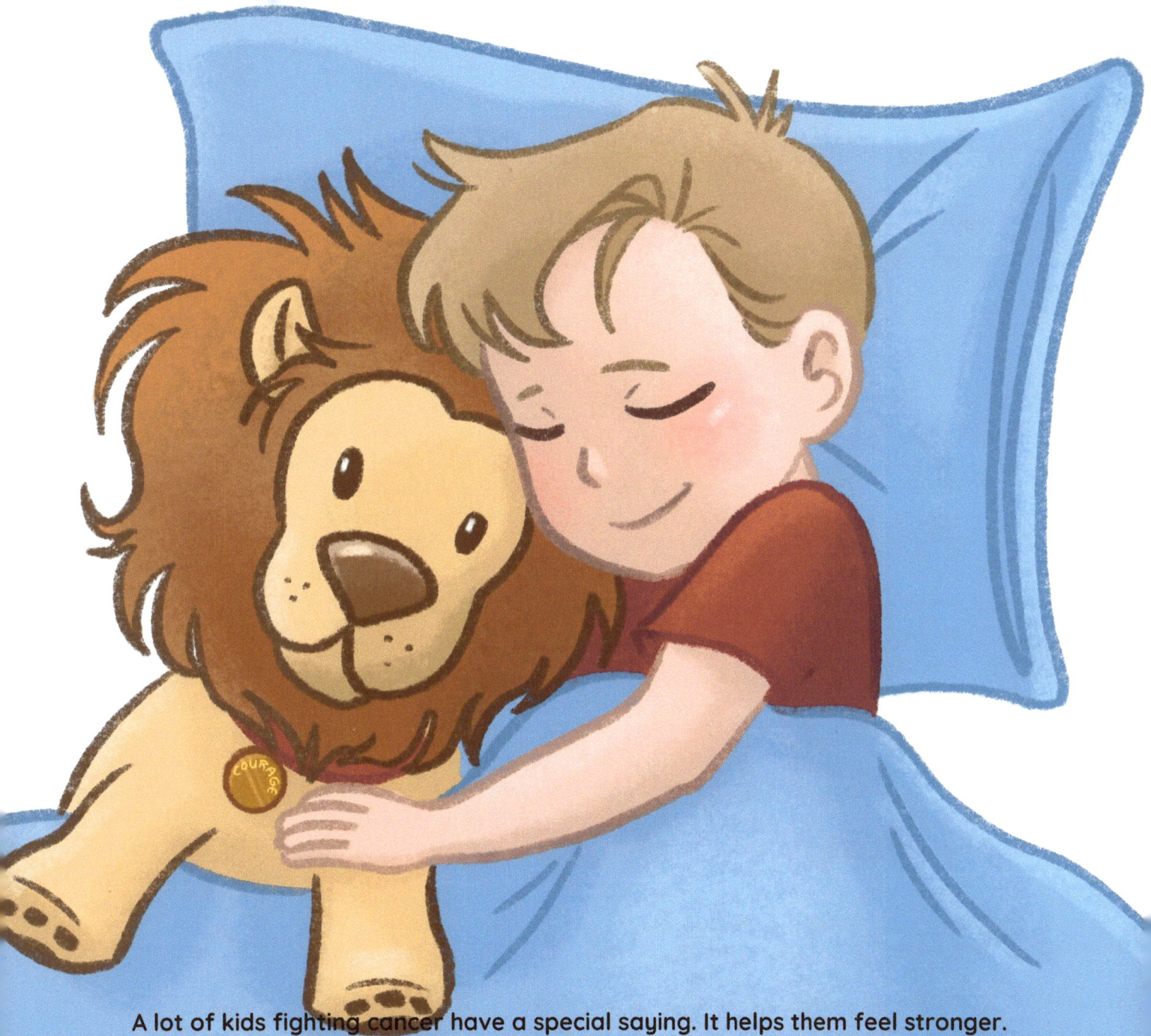

A lot of kids fighting cancer have a special saying. It helps them feel stronger. Mine was "have the courage of a lion". You should come up with one too. It can really inspire you to keep going, even on the hard days.

Something else that kept me going: my family and friends.

They were always there for me. Let your loved ones help you. They want to be by your side, and their love can make a big difference.

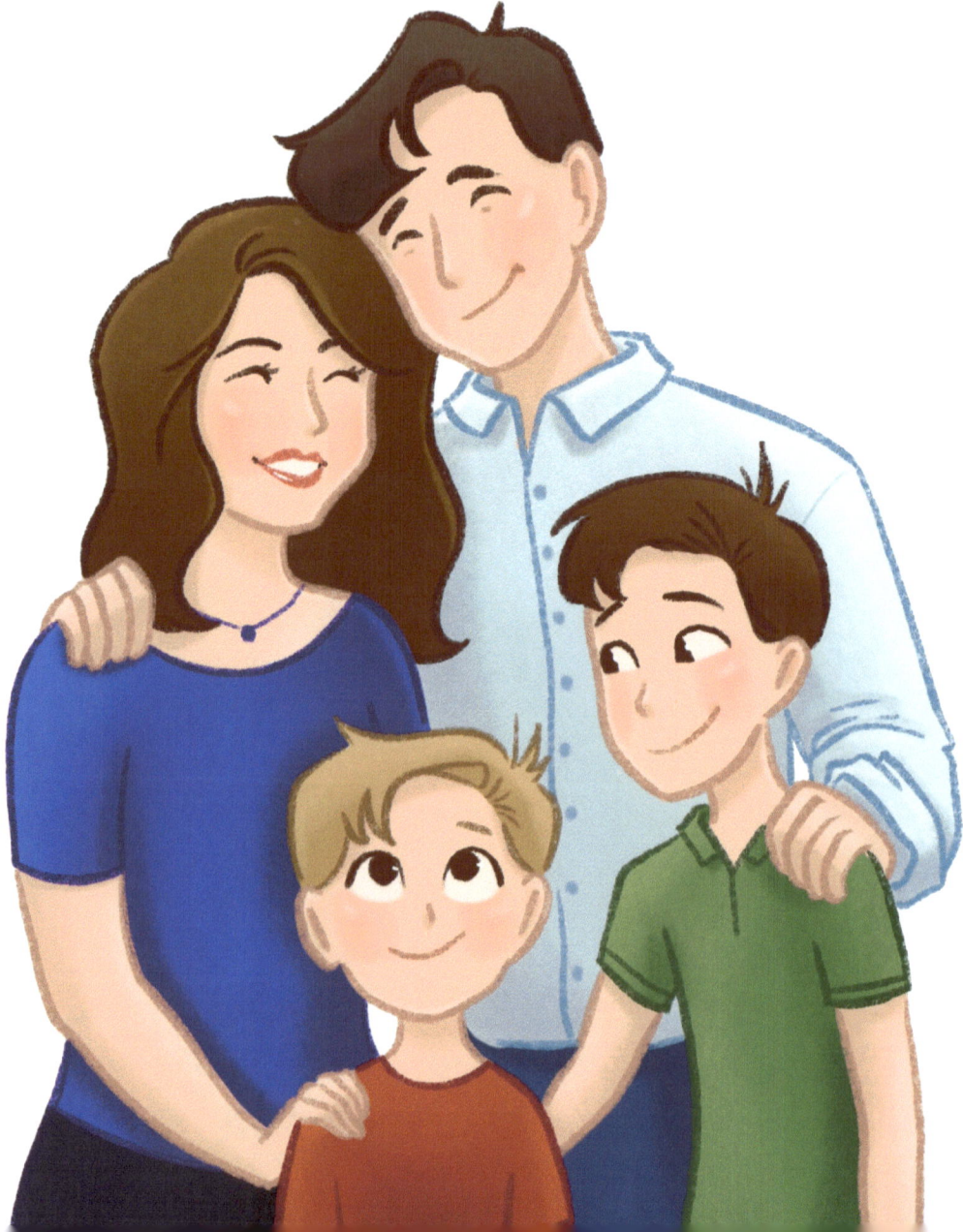

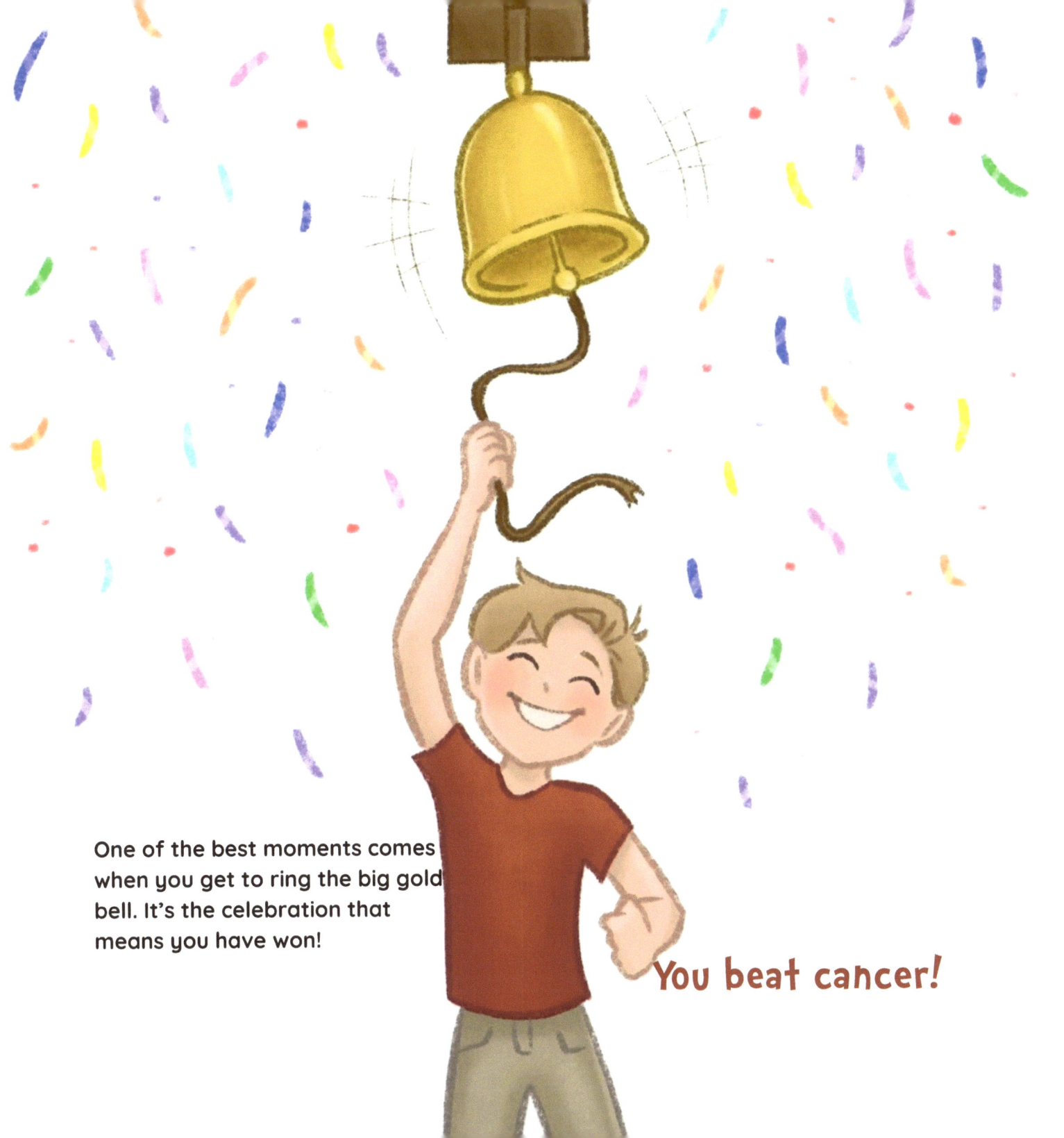

One of the best moments comes when you get to ring the big gold bell. It's the celebration that means you have won!

You beat cancer!

With All My Gratitude

There are people in life who don't just save you, they shape you. Dr. ZoAnn Dreyer and the medical team at Texas Children's Hospital are those people for me. They walked me through some of the hardest moments of my life. As a child facing cancer, I was scared, but never alone. They treated me with compassion and always gave me hope. Today, I am alive, thriving, and forever grateful. I even ran a marathon this year... 26.2 miles!

The photos on the next two pages remind me of where I've been and who helped me get here. From a little boy in a hospital gown to a young man chasing dreams, I carry them with me every step of the way. Thank you for believing in me and fighting for me.

Also, a special shout-out to my elementary school, Cornerstone Christian Academy. They constantly prayed for me, and some faculty and students even shaved their heads to honor what I was going through.

My loving family helped me every step of the way.

A special thanks to Mrs. Tammy McDonald, who came out of retirement to become my kindergarten homeschool teacher and taught me how to write. Also, thank you to Heather Mize, who created my lion mantra, and Bridget Roth, who started my blog, Caleb's Courage.

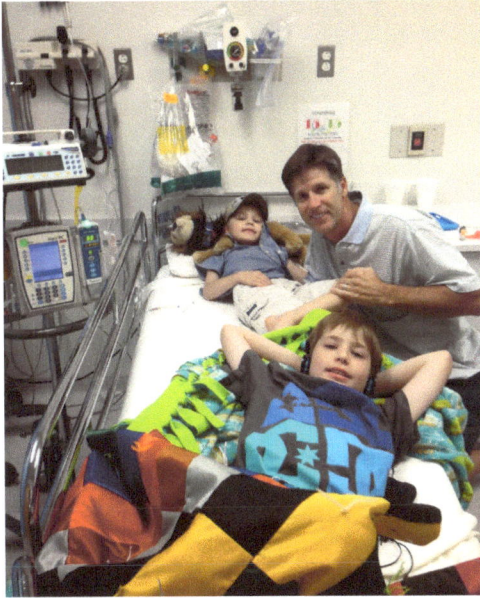
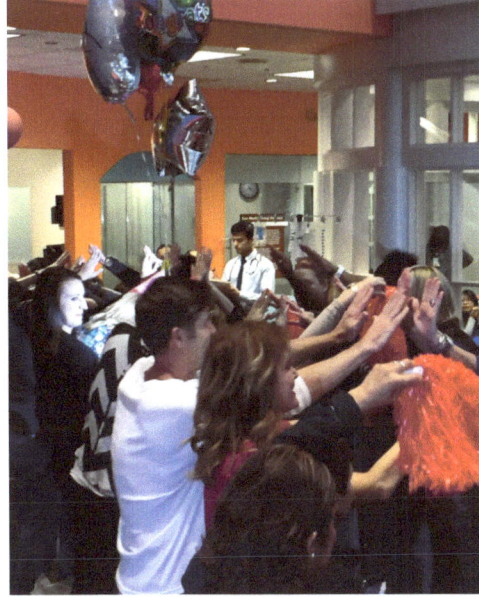
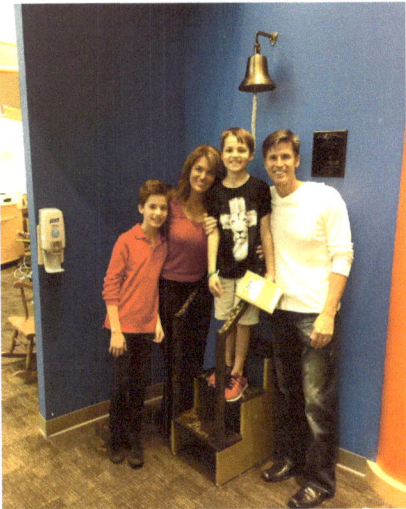
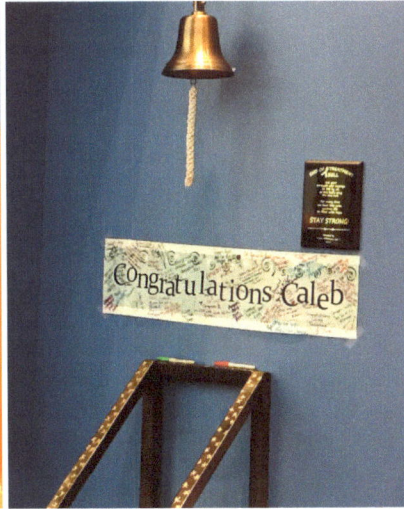
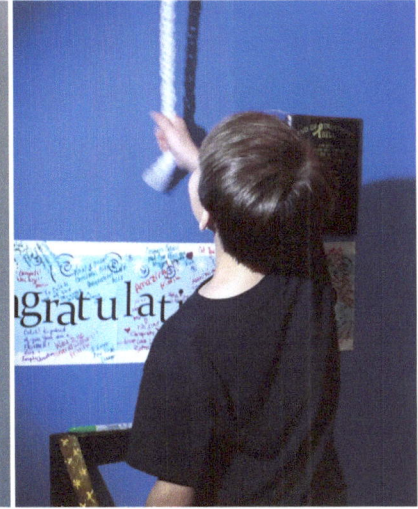

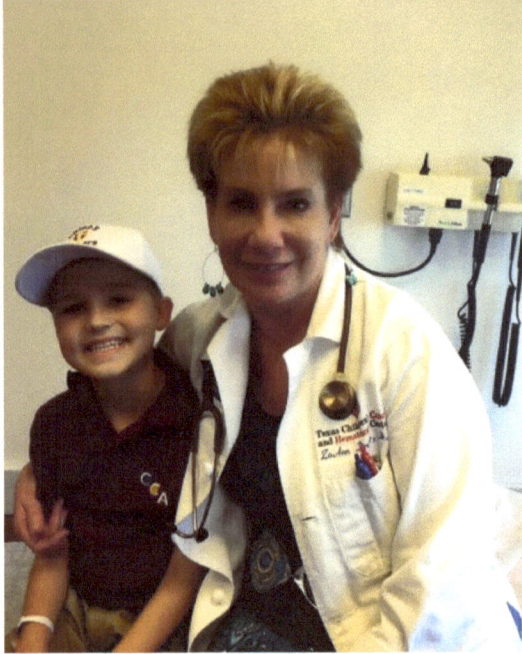
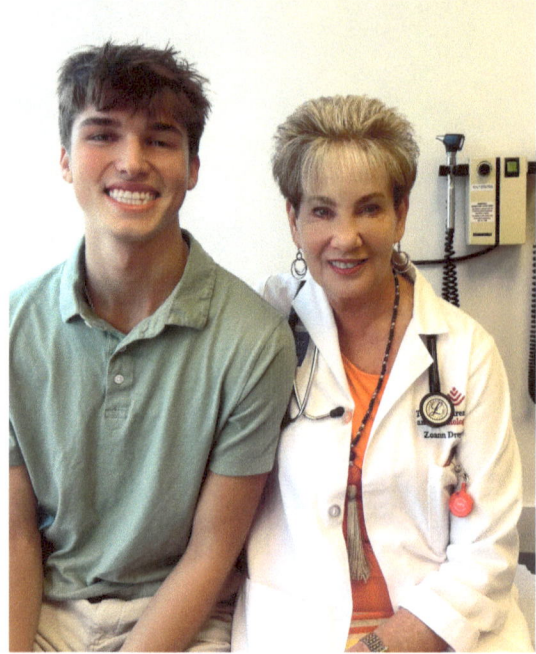

www.ingramcontent.com/pod-product-compliance
Lightning Source LLC
Chambersburg PA
CBHW060853270326
41934CB00002B/121